Psychiatry for Nurses

Psychiatry for Nurses

As per the Syllabus of INC for BSc Students

Second Edition

S Nambi MBBS MD (Psychiatry) DPM
Professor and Head
Department of Psychiatry
Sree Balaji Medical College and Hospital
Chennai, Tamil Nadu, India
Past President
Indian Psychiatric Society
Former Professor
Department of Psychiatry
Madras Medical College/Institute of Mental Health
Chennai, Tamil Nadu, India

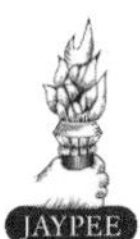

JAYPEE BROTHERS MEDICAL PUBLISHERS
The Health Sciences Publisher
New Delhi | London

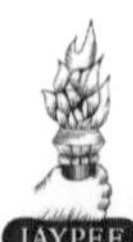

Jaypee Brothers Medical Publishers (P) Ltd

Headquarters
Jaypee Brothers Medical Publishers (P) Ltd
23/23-B, Ansari Road, Daryaganj
New Delhi 110 002, India
Phone: +91-11-23272143, +91-11-23272703
+91-11-23282021, +91-11-23245672
E-mail: jaypee@jaypeebrothers.com

Corporate Office
Jaypee Brothers Medical Publishers (P) Ltd.
4838/24, Ansari Road, Daryaganj
New Delhi 110 002, India
Phone: +91-11-43574357
Fax: +91-11-43574314
E-mail: jaypee@jaypeebrothers.com

Overseas Office
JP Medical Ltd
83 Victoria Street, London
SW1H 0HW (UK)
Phone: +44 20 3170 8910
E-mail: info@jpmedpub.com

EU GPSR Authorised Representative
Logos Europe, 9 rue Nicolas Poussin
17000, La Rochelle, France
Phone: +33 (0) 6 67 93 73 78
E-mail: Contact@logoseurope.eu

Website: www.jaypeebrothers.com
Website: www.jaypeedigital.com

Inquiries for bulk sales may be solicited at: jaypee@jaypeebrothers.com

Psychiatry for Nurses

First Edition: 1998
Reprint: 2002, 2003, 2005, 2006
Second Edition: 2014
ISBN 978-93-5152-379-6

Printed at: Sterling Graphics Pvt. Ltd. India

Dedicated to

The Suffering Mentally Ill Persons

Preface to the Second Edition

The first edition of *Psychiatry for Nurses* published in 1998 had a very good response from both the faculty and students of nursing schools, colleges and that is the reason why four more reprints have been made so far.

The second edition of *Psychiatry for Nurses* maintains a strong student focus presenting sound nursing theory, therapeutic needs and clinical applications. The chapters are short and simple in order to facilitate reading comprehension and student learning. This new edition is supported with few more new chapters like Mental Health Nursing of Disasters, Stigma and Mental Illnesses.

Some of the chapters like Community Psychiatry provides a comprehensive account of District Mental Health Program in India, Treatment of Mental Disorders gives much details about the newer psychotropic drugs and their side effects profile, and in the Legal Aspects of Psychiatric Nursing gives addition of new information about the ensuing Mental Health Care Act, 2013 with changes in the admission procedures. Hence, this second edition provides more comprehensive learning of mental health nursing for nursing students.

In preparing this second edition, I thank My wife Dr Shanthi Nambi, Professor of Child Psychiatry, Madras Medical College for her continuous support and encouragement for assisting me in this task and my Department Assistant Professors Dr Priya and Dr Siva Elango have contributed much and my sincere thanks to them.

I sincerely thank my secretary Ms J Sujatha. Without her help and assistance, I would not have completed this task.

I also express my gratitude to Shri Jitendar P Vij (Group Chairman), Mr Ankit Vij (Group President) and Mr Tarun Duneja (Director-Publishing) and Ms Samina Khan (Executive Assistant to Director-Publishing) of M/s Jaypee Brothers Medical Publishers (P) Ltd, New Delhi, India for all the help they have extended to me for publishing this book.

S Nambi

Preface to the First Edition

'Care of the human mind is the most noble branch of medicine'

Stress of modern life and rapid social changes, accelerated by modern technological achievements, have powerful effects on people's mental health and the quality of their life.

Psychiatric nursing has emerged as a specialized branch of nursing in the recent past in India. Psychiatric training for nurses is essential not only to manage the severely mentally ill or psychotic patients but also to so many other psychological problems which include depression, anxiety and other neurotic disorders, psychosomatic disorders, problems due to alcohol and drug dependence, emotional problems of children, adolescents and elderly population. Apart from these, patients suffering from physical illnesses are also having associated emotional problems, because of the intimate relationship of the body and the mind. The nurse should be able to recognize and take care of these mental health problems. It requires knowledge and application of technical skills.

This book *Psychiatry for Nurses* is written basically for nursing students, who are undergoing training in Mental Health Nursing and who have to write in their examination about psychiatry and psychiatric nursing. This book may also be useful for nurses who work with the mentally ill people in different set-ups like general hospital psychiatric departments, psychiatric hospitals and nursing homes, and in community mental health programs. The purpose of this book is to present a clear and concise account of the common mental health problems, their management and nursing care. The important aim of this book is to introduce nursing students a theoretical and practical approach of the care of the mentally disturbed persons. A sincere attempt has been made in this book to organize current practice of psychiatric nursing so as to enable the nurses to develop an understanding of the complexity of human behavior and the treatment designed to alter adaptive behavior. The chapters in this book are formulated on the syllabus recommended by the Nursing Council of India for the diploma and degree students of nursing. The nursing students can confidently face their psychiatric nursing examination and manage the emotionally disturbed patients more effectively with the help of this book.

I am indebted to the Director, Institute of Mental Health, Chennai, for his support and encouragement to write this book. I extend my thanks to my wife Dr Shanthi Nambi, who has provided the essential assistance. I also thank Ms MR Vijayalakshmi and Mr Ananda Padmanaban, for their secretarial assistance. My sincere thanks to M/s Jaypee Brothers Medical Publishers (P) Ltd, for publishing this book.

S Nambi

Contents

Syllabus

Placement: Third Year

Time: Theory— 90 Hours
Practical—270 Hours
Internship: 95 hours (2 Weeks)

Course Description: This course is designed for developing an understanding of the modern approach to mental health, identification, prevention and nursing management of common mental health problems with special emphasis on therapeutic interventions for individuals, family and community.

Unit	Time (Hrs)	Learning Objective	Content	Teaching Learning Activity	Assessment Method
I	5	• Describes the historical development and current trends in mental health nursing • Describe the epidemiology of mental health problems • Describe the National Mental Health Act, programs and mental health policy • Discusses the scope of mental health nursing • Describe the concept of normal and abnormal behavior	**Introduction** • Perspectives of mental health and mental health nursing: evolution of mental health services, treatments and nursing practices. • Prevalence and incidence of mental health problems and disorders • Mental Health Act • National Mental Health Policy vis a vis National Health Policy • National Mental Health Program • Mental health team • Nature and scope of mental health nursing • Role and functions of mental health nurse in various settings and factors affecting the level of nursing practice • Concepts of normal and abnormal behavior	• Lecture discussion	• Objective type • Short answer • Assessment of the field visit reports

Contd...

Contd...

Unit	Time (Hrs)	Learning Objective	Content	Teaching Learning Activity	Assessment Method
I	5	• Defines the various terms used in mental health nursing • Explains the classification of mental disorders • Explain psychodynamics of maladaptive behavior • Discuss the etiological factors, psychopathology of mental disorders • Explain the principles and standards of mental health nursing • Describe the conceptual models of mental health nursing	**Principles and concepts of mental health nursing** • Definition: Mental health nursing and terminology used • Classification of mental disorders: ICD • Review of personality development, defense mechanisms • Maladaptive behavior of individuals and groups: stress, crisis and disaster(s) • Etiology: Biopsycho-social factors • Psychopathology of mental disorders: Review of structure and function of brain, limbic system and abnormal neurotransmission • Principles of mental health nursing • Standards of mental health nursing practice • Conceptual models and the role of nurse: – Existential model – Psychoanalytical models – Behavioral model – Interpersonal model	• Lecture discussion • Explain using charts • Review of personality development	• Essay type • Short answer • Objective type
III	8	• Describe nature, purpose and process of assessment of mental health status	**Assessment of mental health status** • History taking • Mental status examination • Mini-mental status examination • Neurological examination: Review • Investigations: Related blood chemistry, EEG, CT & MRI	• Lecture discussion • Demon-stration • Practice session • Clinical practice	• Short answer • Objective type • Assessment of skills with check list

Contd...

Contd...

Unit	Time (Hrs)	Learning Objective	Content	Teaching Learning Activity	Assessment Method
			• Psychological tests role and responsibilities of nurse		
IV	6	• Identify therapeutic communication techniques • Describe therapeutic relationship • Describe therapeutic impasse and its intervention	**Therapeutic communication and nurse-patient relationship** • Therapeutic communication: Types, techniques, characteristics • Types of relationship, • Ethics and responsibilities • Elements of nurse patient contract • Review of technique of IPR-Johari Window • Goals, phases, tasks, therapeutic techniques • Therapeutic impasse and its intervention	• Lecture discussion • Demon-stration • Role play • Process recording	• Short answer • Objective type
V	14	• Explain treatment modalities and therapies used in mental disorders and role of the nurse	**Treatment modalities and therapies used in mental disorders** • Psychopharmacology • Psychological therapies: Therapeutic community, psychotherapy-Individual: psycho-analytical, cognitive and supportive, family, group, behavioral, play, psychodrama, music, dance, recreational and light therapy, relaxation therapies: Yoga, meditation, biofeedback • Alternative systems of medicine • Occupational therapy • Physical therapy: Electroconvulsive therapy • Geriatric considerations • Role of nurse in above therapies	• Lecture discussion • Demon-stration • Group work • Practice session • Clinical practice	• Essay type • Short answers • Objective type

Contd...

Contd...

Unit	Time (Hrs)	Learning Objective	Content	Teaching Learning Activity	Assessment Method
VI	5	• Describe the etiology, psychopathology, clinical manifestations, diagnostic criteria and management of patients with schizophrenia, and other psychotic disorders	**Nursing management of patient with schizophrenia, and other psychotic disorders** • Classification: ICD • Etiology, psycho-pathology, types, clinical manifestations, diagnosis • Nursing assessment-history, physical and mental assessment • Treatment modalities and nursing management of patients with schizophrenia and other psychotic disorders • Geriatric considerations • Follow-up and home care and rehabilitation	• Lecture discussion • Case discussion • Case presentation • Clinical practice	• Essay type • Short answers • Assessment of patient management problems
VII	5	• Describe the etiology, psychopathology, clinical manifestations, diagnostic criteria and management of patients with mood disorders	**Nursing management of patient with mood disorders** • Mood disorders: Bipolar affective disorder, mania depression and dysthymia, etc. • Etiology, psychopathology, clinical manifestations, diagnosis, • Nursing assessment-history, physical and mental assessment • Treatment modalities and nursing management of patients with mood disorders • Geriatric considerations • Follow-up and home care and rehabilitation	• Lecture discussion • Case discussion • Case presentation • Clinical practice	• Essay type • Short answers • Assessment of patient management problems

Contd...

Contd...

Unit	Time (Hrs)	Learning Objective	Content	Teaching Learning Activity	Assessment Method
VIII	8	• Describe the etiology, psychopathology, clinical manifestations, diagnostic criteria and management of patients with neurotic, stress related and somatization disorders	**Nursing management of patient with neurotic, stress related and somatization disorders** • Anxiety disorder, phobias, dissociation and conversion disorder, obsessive compulsive disorder, somatoform disorders, post-traumatic stress disorder • Etiology, psychopathology, clinical manifestations, diagnosis • Nursing assessment-history, physical and mental assessment • Treatment modalities and nursing management of patients with neurotic, stress related and somatization disorders • Geriatric considerations • Follow-up and home care and rehabilitation	• Lecture discussion • Case discussion • Case presentation • Clinical practice	• Essay type • Short answers • Assessment of patient management problems
IX	5	• Describe the etiology, psychopathology, clinical manifestations, diagnostic criteria and management of patients with substance use disorders	**Nursing management of patient with substance use disorders** • Commonly used psychotropic substance: Classification, forms, routes, action, intoxication and withdrawal • Etiology of dependence: Tolerance, psychological and physical dependence, withdrawal syndrome, diagnosis, • Nursing assessment-history, physical, mental assessment and drug assay	• Lecture discussion • Case discussion • Case presentation • Clinical practice	• Essay type • Short answers • Assessment of patient management problems

Contd...

Contd...

Unit	Time (Hrs)	Learning Objective	Content	Teaching Learning Activity	Assessment Method
			• Treatment (detoxification, antabuse and narcotic antagonist therapy and harm reduction) and nursing management of patients with substance use disorders • Geriatric considerations • Follow-up and home care and rehabilitation		
X	4	• Describe the etiology, psychopathology, clinical manifestations, diagnostic criteria and management of patients with personality, sexual and eating disorders	**Nursing management of patient with personality, sexual and eating disorders** • Classification of disorders • Etiology, psycho-pathology, character-istics, diagnosis • Nursing assessment-history, physical and mental assessment • Treatment modalities and nursing manage-ment of patients with personality, sexual and eating disorders • Geriatric considerations • Follow-up and home care and rehabilitation	• Lecture discussion • Case discussion • Case presentation • Clinical practice	• Essay type • Short answers • Assessment of patient management problems
XI	6	• Describe the etiology, psychopathology, clinical manifestations, diagnostic criteria and management of childhood and adolescent disorders including mental deficiency	**Nursing management of childhood and adolescent disorders including mental deficiency** • Classification • Etiology, psycho-pathology, characteristics, diagnosis • Nursing assessment-history, physical, mental and IQ assessment • Treatment modalities and nursing management of childhood disorders including mental deficiency	• Lecture discussion • Case discussion • Case presentation • Clinical practice	• Essay type • Short answers • Assessment of patient management problems

Contd...

Contd...

Unit	Time (Hrs)	Learning Objective	Content	Teaching Learning Activity	Assessment Method
			• Follow-up and home care and rehabilitation		
XII	5	Describe the etiology, psychopathology, clinical manifestations, diagnostic criteria and management of organic brain disorders	**Nursing management of organic brain disorders** • Classification: ICD? • Etiology, psycho-pathology, clinical features, diagnosis and differential diagnosis (Parkinson's and Alzheimer's) • Nursing assessment-history, physical, mental and neurological assessment • Treatment modalities and nursing manage-ment of organic brain disorders • Geriatric considerations • Follow-up and home care and rehabilitation	• Lecture discussion • Case discussion • Case presentation • Clinical practice	• Essay type • Short answers • Assessment of patient management problems
XIII	6	Identify psychiatric emergencies and carry out crisis intervention	**Psychiatric emergencies and crisis intervention** • Types of psychiatric emergencies and their management • Stress adaptation model: Stress and stressor, coping, resources and mechanism • Grief: Theories of grieving process, principles, techniques of counseling • Types of crisis • Crisis Intervention: Principles, techniques and process • Geriatric considerations role and responsibilities of nurse	• Lecture discussion • Demon-stration, • Practice session • Clinical practice	• Short answers • Objective type

Contd...

Contd...

Unit	Time (Hrs)	Learning Objective	Content	Teaching Learning Activity	Assessment Method
XIV	4	Explain legal aspects applied in mental health settings and role of the nurse	**Legal issues in mental health nursing** • The Mental Health Act, 1987: Act, Sections, Articles and their implications, etc. • Indian Lunacy Act, 1912 • Rights of mentally ill clients • Forensic psychiatry • Acts related to narcotic and psychotropic substances and illegal drug trafficking • Admission and discharge procedures • Role and responsibilities of nurse	• Lecture discussion • Case discussion	• Short answers • Objective type
XV	4	• Describe the model of preventive psychiatry • Describes Community mental health services and role of the nurse	**Community mental health nursing** • Development of community mental health services: • National Mental Health Program • Institutionalization versus deinstitutionalization • Model of preventive psychiatry: Levels of prevention • Mental health services available at the primary, secondary, tertiary levels including rehabilitation and role of nurse • Mental health agencies: Government and voluntary, national and international • Mental health nursing issues for special populations: Children, adolescence, women, elderly, victims of violence and abuse, handicapped, HIV/AIDS, etc.	• Lecture discussion • Clinical/field practice • Field visits to mental health service agencies	• Short answers • Objective type • Assessment of the field visit reports

Chapter

1

Introduction to Psychiatric Nursing

"Health is not merely the absence of disease but a sense of physical, psychological and social well being". Physical and mental health are like two sides of a coin and both are interdependent. A nurse who is responsible for total health care of a person must take care of the emotional aspect also. The nurse should develop a basic understanding and skill in psychiatric nursing to achieve total health care. She should learn to care for patients with varying degrees of personality deviation and she should understand her role in contributing to positive mental health. This step will enable her to exercise effectively in all areas of nursing.

NEED FOR PSYCHIATRIC NURSING

Psychiatric nursing concepts are an integral part of general nursing. Every nurse who performs the simplest nursing duty gives the patient some psychiatric nursing care whether she is aware of it or not. For example, giving medication. What is important in the nursing role includes not only her knowledge of the properties of the drug, and methods of administration, correct dosage, but also what and how she explains to the patient when giving the drugs and how the patient reacts to it.

1. Psychiatric nursing makes a nurse aware of what she is doing to a patient psychologically.
2. It educates her how to observe her patient.
3. It equips her with appropriate techniques to meet the patient's psychological needs and manage the nurse-patient relationship.

Psychiatric training for nurses is essential not only to manage the severely mentally ill or psychotic patients in psychiatric wards or hospitals, which forms only a part or group, but psychiatric nursing concerns itself with the care of the psychiatric patients extending beyond the walls of the psychiatric hospital to encompass the needs of the family and of the community. She may also have to work in a general hospital that has a psychiatric department/ward. Apart from major mental illnesses, there are many other common psychological problems which include depression, anxiety and other neurotic disturbances, psychosomatic disorders, problems due to alcohol and drug abuse, emotional problems of children, adolescents and elderly population.

Apart from these psychiatric disorders, every medical or surgical condition is accompanied by some emotional problem. The nurse who spends her considerable time with the patient cannot afford to ignore this aspect of the illness. Often patients suffer more from their psychological problems than actual physical pain. Because of the intimate relationship of the body and mind, it is difficult for anything to affect the body without affecting the mind.

The broad principles of psychiatric nursing can thus be applied to patients with medical, surgical, obstetric, orthopedic, pediatrics and psychosomatic conditions as well as patients suffering from neurosis, psychosis, personality disorder and drug dependence.

ROLE OF A NURSE IN THE CARE OF THE PSYCHOLOGICALLY ILL

More usually the nurse acts as a part of a therapeutic team, where, in addition to her traditional work, she has the opportunity to take an active part in other aspects of treatment. Her job is to work with the team to enable each patient get better and return back to the community.

The following are some important tasks of a nurse in a psychiatric set-up.

1. The nurse often has the opportunity to **intervene a behavior** problem on the spot which if ignored or allowed to continue would aggravate the patient's psychological condition.
2. The nurse should conduct brief **counseling** with patients and their families. Such counseling may be formally structured or may take place in informal situations keeping main focus on helping the patients in communicating more clearly.
3. The **technical aspects of patient-care** represent another major role of the nurse. She manages the distribution of drugs, carries out medical treatment and assists in physical methods of treatment.
4. **Reporting** is another main task. The nurse has to record, assess and report to the psychiatrist her observations regarding the patient's behavior, the interaction between the patient and members of his family, the effects of drugs and other forms of treatment, the patient's physical status, etc.
5. The nurse plays the **role of a surrogate mother** when she takes care of the activities of daily living. She keeps him clean, helps him in

the elimination, exercises his inactive limb, and makes sure that he gets sufficient nourishment by well-balanced diet. Exploiting this relationship to the fullest can result in considerable therapeutic benefit to the patient.

6. **Health education** is another important role. The nurse helps patients learn physical and mental hygiene.
7. The nurse **motivates** the patient to participate actively in **rehabilitation programs** like occupational therapy, industrial therapy and recreation therapy.
8. The nurse in a psychiatric set-up also guides and **supervises the functions of other paramedical personnel** in the ward. These staff members work closely with the patients and depend on the nurse for directions and guidance.
9. The nurse as a helping and caring person makes the patient feel supported and reassured. Thus, the nurse acts as a **psychotherapist**. Nurses also conduct family therapy and group therapy in a co-therapist situation or alone or as part of a team. Nursing role in crisis intervention and suicide prevention is very vital.
10. A psychiatric nurse has to play different roles according to the setting. Her job may be looking after demented elderly inpatients at one set-up and working in a therapeutic community run for adolescents in another. Other varied situations include the acute admission ward of a large psychiatric hospital, community work, where patients are seen in their own homes, attachment to a psychiatric department in a general hospital, administrative work, and work in a day hospital or out-patient clinic.

Thus, in the care of the psychologically ill, the nurse has many roles to play. She is:

1. An assistant
2. A caretaker
3. Well-wisher
4. Listener
5. Observer
6. Therapist
7. Motivator
8. Teacher
9. Surrogate mother
10. Administrator
11. Healer.

NURSING ROLE-DIFFERENCE BETWEEN PSYCHIATRIC SET-UP AND OTHER MEDICAL SET-UP

1. The nurse does more for a patient physically in medical or surgical nursing, but in a psychiatric nursing she has to be psychologically active, but physically passive much of the time, listening to an emotionally disturbed patient with pain in his mind may be profoundly touching.
2. In taking care of physical illnesses, the signs and symptoms are generalized and mostly uniform in all patients.
   However in psychiatric patients, for the same disease, the symptoms may vary from individual to individual depending on the nature of the disease, the individual's personality and complex psychobiosocial implications.
3. Physically ill patients respond to the reassurance given by the nurse they are satisfied with the care they are getting and cooperate during the treatment program.
   Emotional disturbance make many psychiatric patients fail to respond to ordinary reassurance in the beginning, because of impaired human relationships these patients often show reactions like mistrust, suspicion and hostility. Patients suffering from major mental illnesses lack insight. They are not aware that they are ill. Hence, they may not cooperate fully during the treatment program. It requires special skills and experience for a nurse to work with such patient.

Chapter

2

Development of Psychiatric Care

Mental illness has been recognized from the earliest times. For many centuries, the mentally ill were among the most tragic examples of man's inhumanity to man. Their behavior, sometimes bizarre, sometimes violent, caused their fellowmen to regard them with suspicion or even outright hostility. At best, the mentally ill were treated with indifference, at worst with cruelty. The mentally ill had to pay a heavy price for their disease.

In early Christian times, mental illness was considered to be the result of possession by demons or evil spirits. The treatment then was to exorcist the demons by prayer, magic, etc. If such treatment brought no improvement, more extreme measures were taken, like punishing them by flogging, burning and even stoning them to death. During this period, the treatment of the mentally ill was in the hands of the priests, who had the power to perform the exorcism.

The first progress in understanding mental disorders came with the Greek physician Hippocrates (460–377 BC). Hippocrates rejected the idea of demonology and maintained that mental disorders were the result of a disturbance in the balance of body fluids. He and other physicians stressed the importance of pleasant surroundings, exercise, proper diet, massage, soothing baths and some less desirable methods such as bleeding, purging and mechanical restraints. Although, there were no institutions for the mentally ill, many were cared for with great kindness by physicians in temples dedicated to Greek and Roman Gods.

Such progress was shortlived, however, the middle ages saw a growing revival of primitive superstition. The mentally ill were thought to be possessed by Satan and supernatural causes. The mentally ill again started getting cruel treatment. Measures such as heating, starving and branding with hot irons were taken against them. The insane were imprisoned, chained and even killed during 15th to 17th centuries.

EARLY ASYLUMS

In the later part of the middle ages, asylums were created. These were not treatment centers, but prisons. The inmates were chained in dark and filthy cells, and treated like animals. In 1792, Philippe Pinel, a French physician unchained these mentally ill against great odds. Pinel's experiment was a success and mentally ill was given better living conditions and started receiving kind treatment.

The turn of this century brought great changes in medicine and psychology. The discovery of spirochetes which caused syphilis in 1905 demonstrated that there was a physical cause for the mental disorder, and encouraged physicians to believe that mental illness was organic in origin.

The work of Sigmund Freud and his followers laid the basis for the understanding of mental illness as a malfunction of the mind and environmental factors. Pavlov's learning theory made a great impact in modifying abnormal behavior.

Despite these developments in the early part of the century, mental hospitals and mental patients were still considered as objects of fear and horror. In the early 1930, Insulin coma therapy originated, where a dose of insulin large enough to produce unconsciousness was given. Some patients improved by this method.

Electroconvulsive therapy was first used by Cerletti and Bini in 1938 to treat mental illness. It proved to be a highly successful treatment and is still used today.

Until the mid 1950s, there were few drugs which could be used effectively in the treatment of mental illness. Bromide, chloral hydrate and barbiturates were subsequently discovered and used with success. In the early 1950s, the first tranquilizing drug became available. The drug was named chlorpromazine (Largactil) and it had the effect of calming the patient without making him sleep. Since then, a variety of tranquilizers and antidepressants have been manufactured which have revolutionalized the treatment of mentally ill.

New and important discoveries were made in the field of human psychology. Many of these discoveries were applied to the care and treatment of the mentally ill. Among the best known was Freud's psychoanalysis, which threw new light on the functioning of the mind in health and sickness. Many psychological methods of treatment like psychotherapy, behavior therapy, family therapy, therapeutic community and cognitive therapy came into existence, and have been a great help in managing the mentally disturbed. In the last few decades, there has been tremendous progress in understanding the biology of behavior and there are many researches going on around the world relating to psychiatric disorders. The genetic influence of mental disorders has been recognized. The biochemical bases for many disorders have already been discovered or are being studied. Such developments in Biological Psychiatry will tremendously influence psychiatric care in the future.

THE FUNCTIONS OF A MODERN PSYCHIATRIC HOSPITAL

The modern psychiatric hospital has four fundamental functions. With partial hospitalization, a person may spend the day in the hospital receiving treatment and return home in the evening (day hospital) or work during the day and spend nights at the hospital (night hospital). Such a program has great flexibility.

A hospital which provides treatment for the mentally ill allows freedom of choice and encourages patients to participate in their own treatment. It is often referred to as a therapeutic community. In a modern psychiatric hospital, patients are treated, helped and encouraged by a therapeutic team. This team consists of psychiatrists, psychologists, nurses, social workers, occupational therapists and other paramedical professionals. Psychiatrists are doctors of medicine, who have special qualifications in psychiatry. Psychiatric nurses are trained to care for the mentally ill. They work closely with the psychiatrist and other members of the team, and are involved in the treatment, care and rehabilitation of the patient. Clinical psychologists are non-medical professionals qualified in understanding the human behavior. They are able to test patients to find the reasons for their behavior. A psychiatric social worker is a part of the mental health-care team. Their work is assessing the detailed history of the patient, analyzing the socioeconomic background and assisting in rehabilitation program. Occupational therapists play an important role in helping patients to relate to others through work and activity.

In addition to these members of the team, there are pharmacists, biochemists, laboratory assistants, recreation therapists, hospital workers, administrative staff and others to organize and carry out the day-to-day running of the hospital.

It is team effort which ultimately makes psychiatric care fruitful and efficient.

HISTORY OF PSYCHIATRIC CARE IN INDIA

Towards the end of 18th Century, lunatic asylums were established in three Presidencies in India—Calcutta, Madras and Bombay. The lunatic asylum in Calcutta was established some time prior to 1787. The one in Madras was set up in 1794 by Dr Valentine Connolly. The Bombay asylum was established in 1858. The lunatic asylums were initially meant for the safe custody of the mentally ill; gradually they started giving care and treatment. In the beginning of the 19th century, these asylums were called mental hospitals. Thus, from mere custodial places they became treatment centers.

The Madras Mental Hospital (now the Institute of Mental Health) is one of the oldest and largest in South-East Asia. It celebrated its 200 years of service to the mentally ill in 1994. At present, there are around 50 mental hospitals in India, with bed strength of 25,000. In general hospital psychiatric units, there are around 5000 beds available for psychiatric patients. All the government-run medical colleges in India have a full-fledged psychiatric department. There are nearly 5000 qualified psychiatrists at present in the country.

One of the significant developments in psychiatry in India, during the last three decades is the establishment of psychiatry units in general hospitals promoting community psychiatry. This has lead to an increased interaction between the psychiatrists and clinicians from other specialties and the development of Consultation-Liaison Psychiatry. There has also been the implementation of the District Mental Health Program (DMHP) under National Mental Health Program to cater to the need of the underprivileged rural population.

Chapter 3

The Process and Development of Psychiatric Nursing

Psychiatric nursing has been recognized as a profession after a long struggle. There are two basic needs in psychiatric nursing:

Defining the nursing.

Identifying a scientific method for delivery of nursing.

DEFINITION OF NURSING

"Nursing is the diagnosis and treatment of human responses to actual or potential health problems" (American Nurses Association 1980).

Thus, the emphasis is on problematic, psychosocial and behavioral human responses of patients rather than upon diagnostic categories of mental illness, which are diagnosed and treated by psychiatrists.

The Nursing Process has been identified as the Nurse's Scientific Methodology for the delivery of nursing care. The curriculum of all nursing schools and colleges, as per the recommendation of the Indian Nursing Council, now includes psychiatric nursing as a component of their conceptual framework.

Nursing diagnosis is an integral part of the nursing process, "Nursing diagnosis provides the basis for prescriptions for definitive therapy for which the nurse is accountable (Kim, et al. 1984).

The essential component of psychiatric nursing is the nurse-patient relationship. This relationship being therapeutic in nature has to be developed around the three essential qualities of a therapeutic relationship namely, empathy, warmth and genuineness. Psychiatric nurses should have the ability to utilize these elements in their work. The following are the essential qualities that form the process of psychiatric nursing. (William Reynolds, et al. 1990).

- Recognition and understanding of the elements of the relationship
- Appropriate thinking and problem solving
- Theoretical framework and interactional structure
- Therapeutic use of self.

Questions that relate to nursing behavior in a variety of situations are presented according to the five steps of the nursing process. According to Townsend, (1988), the five steps of the nursing process are:

Assessment Establishing a data base about a patient.
Analysis Identifying the patient's health-care needs and selecting goals of care.
Planning Designing a strategy to achieve the goals established for the patient.
Implementing Initiating and completing actions necessary to accomplish the defined goals.
Evaluating Determining the extent to which the goals have been achieved.

By following these five steps, the nurse has a systematic framework for decision-making and problem-solving in the delivery of nursing care.

THE QUALITIES OF AN IDEAL PSYCHIATRIC NURSE

A nurse working with psychiatric patients should:
- Be sympathetic and understanding
- Have patience and a capacity to listen
- Be a good observer
- Be bold and helpful to the patient
- Have non-judgmental attitude towards the patient's behavior
- Be available during an emotional crisis
- Be confidential.

The following things which a nurse should not do to her psychiatric patients:
- Pass comments
- Laugh at
- Be sarcastic
- Be biased
- Avoid contact
- Let him down
- Label him.

Nursing Notes

Nurses should keep notes about their psychiatric patients. Nursing notes are valuable since they help the psychiatrist to assess the patient's behavioral patterns. The nurse is the one who spends maximum time with the patient in the ward; hence her observations help in understanding the patient better.

The nurse should write relevant notes to help plan, implement and evaluate the patient's therapeutic regime. The purpose of writing nursing reports is primarily to communicate and share information with others who are involved in the welfare of the patient. There should be some goal in her mind when a nurse writes her notes. The nurse should include in her notes, her personal interview with the patient, her observations on the overall behavior and mood of the patient and about problem situations, if any. The nursing notes should be:

Clean and Precise

Use patient's own words when describing specific problems, like delusion and hallucination.

Give specific examples instead of giving her own interpretation and inference.

The notes should answer the four 'Ws', whenever, describing a problem situation, i.e. "Who", "When", "Where", "Why".

DEVELOPMENT OF PSYCHIATRIC NURSING

Psychiatric nursing arose from the need to provide secure and socially acceptable levels of caring for the emotionally disturbed. The first school to train nurses in mental health was opened in 1882 at McLeod Hospital, Waverby, Massachusetts in the United States. The history of psychiatric nursing was written in detail by Hildegard Peplau (1959). She defined psychiatric nursing as belonging to two areas:

A vital skill of general nursing practice used by all nurses.

An area of clinical specialization practiced by those who have a diploma or degree in psychiatric nursing.

There are five stages in the history of psychiatric nursing:

From 1773–1882, psychiatric nursing did not exist as such, but the need was felt. The care was usually custodial and harsh.

From 1882–1914, mental health nurses were trained and introduced into mental health facilities in the West. Methods of treatment and mental hygiene movements were introduced.

From 1915–1935, special psychiatric nursing education in degree level started. The first textbook in this field by a nurse was published in 1920 (Bailey).

Postgraduate psychiatric nursing education developed from **1926–1945.** Psychiatric nursing was also entering the main stream of nursing with the establishment of the mental health and psychiatric nursing projects.

Psychiatric nursing was recognized as an integral part of nursing with representation in major organizations.

The two World Wars provided at least two lessons significant for psychiatric nursing.

More nurses with better training were needed, and more effective short-term treatment for stress-related disorders needed to be developed.

The 1963, Community Mental Health Act in the United States paved way for community mental health centers with the aim of prevention of mental illness at primary, secondary and tertiary levels. Today, psychiatric nursing has emerged as a profession on its own in the West. There was found to be improved clinical practice after the holistic health movement started.

THE PROCESS AND DEVELOPMENT OF PSYCHIATRIC NURSING—HISTORICAL OVERVIEW

Psychiatric Nursing in India

In India, the progress in mental health remains very slow. As mentioned elsewhere in the book, psychiatric nursing education is following the progress of USA to go before the actual care of mentally ill benefits from psychiatric nursing care.

250 BC—Edicts of Ashoka indicates institutional care of mentally ill existed way back as 250 BC.

15th Century AD—A special hospital for mentally ill was established at Dhar in Madhya Pradesh, first asylum, ayurvedic and Unani treatments were practiced.

1917-1950—Psychiatric nursing was mainly carried out by army nurses.

1946—Report of health survey committee nurses to be prepared in psychiatric nursing also. Committee recommended the existing institution like Bangalore and Ranchi Mental Hospital to start training for nursing personnel.

1950—5-8 hours of psychiatry was included in the syllabus, but no examination was conducted or no clinical experience provided.

1956—1 year post-certificate course in psychiatric nursing started at National Institute of Mental Health and Neurosciences (NIMHANS).

1960—Postgraduate diploma in psychiatric nursing started in Ranchi.

1964—Mudaliar Committee recommended preparation of a large number of psychiatric nurses. INC—Nursing curriculum should have a component of psychiatric nursing.

1965—INC—Included psychiatric nursing as a compulsory course in BSc (N) program.

1966—Psychiatric nursing component was added in the general nursing and midwifery (GNM) course.

1975—Psychiatric nursing was offered as elective subject in Msc(N) at Rajkumari Amrit Kaur College of Nursing (RAKCN), New Delhi.

1978—First postgraduate clinically oriented research was conducted and was published in 1968 in the Indian Journal of Psychiatry. First psychiatric nurse whose article was published in a journal.

1980—Practical and oral examinations were made compulsory. 30-35 hours of psychiatry and psychiatric nursing.

1985—50 hours in the curriculum.

1986—Recent revision GNM syllabus content of psychiatric nursing has been dealt within more depth.

1987—The new Mental Health Act.

1990—4 colleges MSc program in psychiatric nursing at Mumbai, Chandigarh, Ludhiana, and Vellore.

2000-2005—Many colleges have Master's level program.

Psychiatry, from the initial mental hospital set-up, where custodial care was the only care, developed into a place where treatment methods were started. Then, it slowly crawled into the general hospital with the formation of separate psychiatric departments. The third stage came when Community Mental Health program is being seriously discussed about after National Mental Health Program in 1982.

During the last 65 years, psychiatry has made spectacular progress and undergone many revolutionary changes in India. Psychiatric nursing has evolved as a recognized specialty area in nursing in the later part of the last century. Significant progress in the psychiatric education for nurses was made between 1945-1960 in the developed countries and after 1960 in India. Two historical events are noteworthy in this regard. First, the introduction and widespread use of psychotropic drugs, especially chlorpromazine in the treatment of mental patients in the 1950s increased the potential for viable treatment and care of the mentally ill. Second was the introduction of a diploma in psychiatric nursing at the National Institute of Mental Health in Bengaluru followed by few centers like Christian Medical College, Vellore. In the later decade, psychiatric nursing has been introduced in the Postgraduate level (MSc) in few centers in India.

Training nursing students in various psychiatric set-ups provides opportunities for further development of a specialty area in nursing that concentrates on the care and treatment of the mentally ill. In the last few years, psychiatric nursing has become an examination subject and there are board and university examinations in psychiatric nursing for both diploma in nursing and degree (BSc) students respectively. Thus, psychiatric nursing has emerged as an essential part of the curriculum of nursing education.

Future of Psychiatric Nursing

Mental health and psychiatric nursing needs to successfully confront two challenges in the future. First, nurses must actively participate in establishing the conditions under which interpersonal treatment methods are effective in preventing and relieving psychiatric disorders. Second, nurses must actively participate in establishing the conditions under which mental health and psychiatric nursing practice interacts with the treatment methods emerging from biological research in preventing or relieving psychiatric disorders.

Chapter

4

Basic Psychology

The sum total of values, attitudes and consistent behavior patterns that are unique to one person is termed as the personality.

Although, the hereditary factors affect personality to some degree, environmental factors are the most important determinants of personality.

Sigmund Freud, the Father of Psychoanalysis, believed that a healthy personality depended on a successful transition through fine psychosexual stages of oral, anal, phallic, latency, and genital each with its particular conflict that must have overcome.

Freud, in his psychoanalytic approach, believed that the early childhood experiences do not disappear without trace. He stated that the mind could be divided into three levels:

The conscious

The preconscious (subconscious), and

The unconscious.

The conscious mind contains all that we are aware of at any given moment.

The subconscious mind comprises of memories, thoughts and feelings, which we are able to bring into consciousness at will.

The unconscious mind contains all the memories, wishes and feelings that we do not know about and cannot recall even if we try. These can be brought out by psychoanalysis.

Psychoanalysis can be processed through two ways:
Free Association, and Dream Analysis.

According to Freud's theory, the personality includes three separate, but interacting systems.

The Id

The Ego, and

The Super Ego.

Id: The primitive unconscious part of the personality. Id is the source of instinctual energy, which works on the pleasure principle. Id seeks complete and immediate gratification of desire.

Ego: Ego is the reality-based aspect of the self. Ego is that part of the personality that seeks to satisfy the Id and the super ego. It is the reality and practical mind.

Super ego: Super ego is the moral branch of mental functioning. It is the controlling mind.

When ego is able to balance between Id and super ego, the mind can function normally. When there is ego disturbance, there is bound to be mental imbalance and problems.

DEFENSE MECHANISMS (MENTAL MECHANISMS)

Sigmund Freud first identified a unique set of emotional coping strategies that he called Ego Defense Mechanisms. Defense mechanism is any automatic, unconscious response that helps a person reduces painful feelings associated with emotional problems.

Characteristics of Defense Mechanisms

They protect the person from anxiety

They protect the person from insult by boosting self-esteem or through self-enhancement.

Defense mechanisms are not used deliberately; rather, they are unconscious or at least partly so.

Defense mechanisms operate by:

- Masking or disguising our true motives
- Denying the existence of impulses, actions or memories within ourselves that might be provoked anxiety to us.

Adaptive mental mechanisms thus protect us from anxiety. All of us at times use defense mechanisms. Defense mechanisms are essential for healthy adaptation. Like anxiety, defense mechanisms can contribute in a positive sense to an individual's development. Through over use or failure when needed, defense mechanisms lead to disruptive and unhappy life patterns.

Common Defense Mechanisms and Their Usage

Repression

Involuntarily forgetting about unacceptable ideas, impulses or events.

Example: A patient had a sudden strong urge to defecate and was incontinent before the nurse could help her on to the bed pan; the patient was extremely embarrassed by the situation, however, a month later the same person had totally forgotten at the incident and did not remember it again.

Sublimation

Channeling or diverting unacceptable feelings into socially approved behavior. Sublimation is a widely used mental mechanism.

Example: The unmarried woman may channel her sexual energy into working for charity or dedication to her job. Aggressive people may channel their energy by playing competitive sports.

Reaction Formation

Unconsciously dealing with unacceptable desires by behaving the opposite way to true feelings

Example

a. A married woman who is disturbed by her attraction to another man may state forcefully that she dislikes him.
b. A patient is afraid of surgery, but instead acts unconcerned about it and jokes about others who are frightened of surgery.

Dissociation

Unconsciously removing painful experiences from the conscious mind.

Example: The man who is unhappily married is unable to remember his married life.

This mental mechanism produces symptoms like hysteria.

Conversion

Unconsciously converting or changing painful feelings or emotions into a bodily symptoms.

Example: The girl who is not willing to marry a man, because she is in love with another person may have a fit a few weeks prior to the marriage.

This mechanism operates in hysteria.

Rationalization

Unconsciously making up or giving excuses for behavior. The person gives acceptable reasons for the things he does and protects himself from the truth.

Example

a. A person who drinks alcohol to derive pleasure or to avoid withdrawal symptoms says that he drinks because his wife nags him.
b. The girl who always wears revealing dresses to party says that she can never find anything else to wear.

Projection

Unconsciously shifting the blame on to other people or circumstances.

Example

a. A poor workman always blames his tools.
b. The demanding, selfish girl will blame her boyfriend and not herself, when he finally jilts her.

Regression

Returning to a childish form of behavior when faced with a distressing situation to relieve anxiety. Regression is generally seen in children, who sometimes return to an earlier stage of development on the arrival of a new baby in the house.

Example: The patient who is extremely anxious about hospital treatment may become completely dependent (like a child) on the nurses refusing to do even the smallest thing for himself.

Chapter

5

The Brain and Behavior

Man has the capacity for thought, and thought is the integrative activity of the brain. Physiological psychology is the study of the relationship between behavior and brain. It has been observed that 'mind' is an integrative capacity developed by the brain. Thinking, decision making, memory, intelligence, emotions, control over one's behavior and talk and awareness of surroundings are all different functions of the mind. Mind is the active part of our 'Self' and is the source of all our activities. The brain carries out all the functions of the mind. The basic unit of the nervous system and the brain is the Neuron. The brain is made up of millions of such nerve cells.

The brain can be divided into three parts.

- Brain stem
- Limbic system
- Cerebral cortex

The Brain stem is responsible for the basic or vital functions of the body like respiration, heart/pulse, blood pressure, consciousness, etc. Damage to the brain stem can lead to loss of consciousness and even death.

The Limbic system controls emotions and sexual behavior. The limbic system lies beneath the cerebral hemispheres and above the central core. Its highly interrelated structures (primarily the hippocampus, the amygdala and the septal area) rig the tip of the brain's central core, connecting with the cerebral cortex, The limbic system is called the emotional brain as it is involved in emotional and goal-directed behavior. It plays a role in feeding, fighting, fleeing and mating. Pleasure centers have been located in the limbic system and the hippocampus appears to have a role in memory.

The cerebral cortex is responsible for thinking, memory, social behavior, speech, language, decision making, perception and other behavior. Different parts of the cerebral cortex are responsible for different functions.

For example, the frontal lobe is for thinking and social behavior, the occipital lobe is related to visual perception; the temporal lobe is involved in hearing and smell and the parietal lobe controls movements of the body and sensory perceptions. The left part of the brain controls thinking, speech, language, ability to master technological issues, while right brain is responsible for the ability to know the position of articles in space, music, dancing and other artistic abilities, emotions and spiritual thinking.

NEUROTRANSMITTERS

Most drugs used in Psychiatry Act by altering neurotransmission. Drugs act either presynaptically to influence levels of the neurotransmitter in the synaptic cleft or postsynaptically by agonist, antagonist or modulatory actions at postsynaptic receptors.

Neurotransmission describes the process by which information is transferred from one neuron to another neuron across the synaptic cleft. Activation of the postsynaptic receptor may result in either:

Excitation—Membrane depolarization or
Inhibition—Membrane hyperpolarization

Neurotransmitter is a chemical substance that helps in the transmission of message from one nerve cell to other. It acts as a bridge and helps the message to reach the other neuron. When an individual thinks, talks, or does anything, many such neurotransmitters are actively involved. When extreme changes occur in the neurotransmitter mechanism, the function of the mind gets disturbed.

The characteristics of a neurotransmitter

- It must be manufactured in the presynaptic terminal of a neuron
- It should be released when a nerve impulse reaches the terminal
- Its presence in the synaptic gap must generate a biological response in the next neuron
- If its release is blocked, there must be no subsequent response.

The following are the common neurotransmitters:

Amines
a. Acetylcholine (ACh)
b. Dopamine (DA)
c. Noradrenaline (NA)
d. Serotonin (5-HT)
e. Histamine

Amino Acids
a. Glutamate
b. GABA (GABA Aminobutyric acid)

Others
a. Enkephalins
b. Beta- endorphins
c. Substance-P
d. Cholecystokinin
e. Neurotensin

Endocannabinoids.

INVOLVEMENT OF NEUROTRANSMITTER IN VARIOUS PSYCHIATRIC DISORDERS

Disorder	*Neurotransmitter*
1. Schizophrenia	Dopamine Glutamate Serotonin
2. Depression	Serotonin Noradrenaline
3. Anxiety disorders	GABA Serotonin
4. Alcohol dependence	GABA
5. Dementia	Acetylcholinesterase

Behavior

Man acquires a number of reflex responses to stimuli known as conditioned reflexes (Pavlov). The sight or smell of food produces salivation in animal (unconditioned response) when a sound of bells frequency associated with food, mere sound of bell before food also (conditioned stimulus) produced salivation (conditioned response) after associated these stimuli with food. This is known as classical conditioning.

Skinner used another type of conditioning called operant or instrumental conditioning. In this conditioning, the positive consequence of an action (reward) itself acts as the conditioning stimulus motivating further response of the same kind.

These two types of conditioning phenomenon underline the paradigms of human learning.

Learning

Learning is the process of modification of response to stimuli. Learning involves growth of new synaptic connections. The simple stimulus response learning is integrated subcortically (involving the reticular formation). Abstract learning and complex forms of learning involve the entire association areas of the neocortex. Ability to learn new information is affected in lesions of these areas particularly the prefrontal cortex.

Memory

Memory is the registration, storage and subsequent recall of learned experiences.

Short-term memory: The first stage of memory is the registration, i.e. processing of sensory input from the very brief immediate past to be held is the short-term memory.

Long-term memory: The second stage of memory is the storage, i.e. conversion of short-term memory to a stable long-term memory. The conversion occurs possibly in the hippocampus. In this conversion, the acoustic coding is transformed into semantic coding. Amnesia is loss of memory. Lesions in hippocampus, mammillary bodies and dorsomedial thalamus produce loss of memory.

Like this, all the human behavior have basis in the neuroanatomy and/or neurophysiology.

Chapter

6

Mental Health

"Health is not merely the absence of disease or infirmity. It is a condition of physical, mental and social wellbeing".

One should strive to attain the highest possible level of health, a level that will permit one to lead a socially and economically productive life.

Mental health does not mean mere absence of mental illness. It is a sense of well-being an individual feels. There should be some positive qualities in every human being that enables him to live happily in society. Mental health and physical health are interrelated and interdependent. As the saying goes, 'A sound mind in a sound body', mental and physical health are the two sides of a coin.

DEFINITION OF MENTAL HEALTH

World Health Organization defines mental health as "the capacity of an individual to form harmonious relationships with others and to participate in, or contribute constructively to changes in the social environment."

Menninger defines Mental Health as "The adjustment of human beings to the world and to each other with a maximum of effectiveness and happiness."

Mental health is an ability to maintain:

An even temper

An alert intelligence

A socially considerate behavior, and

A happy disposition.

Good adjustment is the basic component of mental health. Mental health is an individual and personal matter. It involves an individual human mind. A social environment or culture may be conducive either to sickness or health, but the quality produced is characteristic only of a person. Mental health is a state in which one's potential capacities are fully realized. Maturity, as adjustment, can also be regarded as mental health. The terms 'mature', 'well adjusted' and 'psychologically healthy' are often used as synonyms. There should be a positive approach to attain mental health.

CHARACTERISTICS OF A MENTALLY HEALTHY PERSON

A mentally healthy person is free from internal conflicts. He is not at war with himself.

He is well adjusted. He is able to get along well with others. He is able to form effective relationships. He accepts criticism and is not easily upset.

He searches for an identity.

He has a strong sense of self-esteem.

He knows himself, his needs, problems and goals (This is known as self actualization).

He has good control over his behavior.

He is productive.

He faces problems and tries to solve them intelligently, i.e. he has the ability to cope with stress and anxiety.

Mental health is the full and harmonious functioning of the whole personality. Three requirements of mental health are:

Full expression (of potential, personality, etc.).

Harmonization.

The direction to a common end of our native and acquired potentials.

Living in a stress free environment will pave the way for mentally healthier and happier life. In general, mental health can be achieved in many ways, like individual treatment, treatment of families and educational program. Sound behavior patterns can be encouraged and reinforced in a well established social network. Thus, healthy social surrounding is the need of the hour. Mental health is a positive science as it sets out to establish a condition of healthy mindedness.

MENTAL HEALTH EDUCATION AND MENTAL HEALTH PROGRAMS

Misconception and Public Attitude towards Mental Illness

Following are some of the common misconceptions among the public:

Mental illnesses are caused by Gods as punishment for sin, or by ghosts, black magic, evil powers and witchcraft.

Mental patients are different from other people.

Psychiatric illness is not like physical illness.

Psychiatric patients never get well; once mentally ill, they are always mentally ill.

Psychiatric patients should take drugs throughout their life time.

Psychiatric patients are always violent and dangerous.

Professionals like psychiatrists, psychiatric nurses, who work with the mentally ill persons are likely to become disturbed themselves.

Some of these misconceptions are culturally based. It is the responsibility of the nurse to correct these by providing clarification and information. It cannot be achieved in one day, but with sustained effort it can.

How to Overcome These Prejudices or Attitudes?

Health education (social education) is the answer.

Social education aims at educating the public about mental illnesses. It can be done by:

Making use of media or mass communication.

Conducting public lectures, organizing mental health exhibitions.

Distributing pamphlets.

Group discussions involving selected groups like: teachers, employers, native leaders, etc.

Encouraging the community to visit mental health centers.

Extending psychiatric service to general hospitals.

Demonstrating the usefulness of treatment.

Advising the family to participate in treatment programs.

Chapter

7

Mental Health Services in India

Man is essentially thinking and feeling organism. Therefore, no scheme of health planning can be complete which does not take the mental health component into account. Mental health care is a part of, but not apart from, total health care.

The psychiatric services form a part of the complex health and social services essential for the community wellbeing. Their task is to bring to the public the benefit of available mental health knowledge and skill. The increasing complexity of modem life has added a new dimension to the problem.

For the provision of any Health Care Program, the following four indicators are to be taken into account.

- Availability
- Accessibility
- Utilization, and
- Quality of care.

Magnitude of mental health problem in India:

- Nearly twenty percent of the population suffers from some sort of psychological disturbance
- Nearly one percent of the population suffers from major mental illness. That means around 8–9 million suffer from severe mental disturbances in India
- Around five percent suffer from mood disorders (especially depression)
- Anxiety and other disorders are found in 7–9 percent of the population
- Around 3–5 percent of population suffers from ill-effects of excessive alcohol, drinking and drug addiction
- Dementia is found in four percent of the subjects aged over 60
- In children, nearly 3 percent suffer from some sort of mental retardation and five percent suffer from emotional and conduct disorder
- It is also estimated that around 15–20 percent of people who seek medical help in various Health Care Centers have mild psychological disturbances, but most of them are not aware of it.

Majority of Indian patients with psychiatric disturbance remain without help for long time because of ignorance, fear, stigma, misconception and faulty attitudes regarding mental illnesses. People in our country still believe that mental illnesses are caused by ghosts, evil spirits, black magic, witchcraft, bad stars and sins. Therefore, they seek the help of faith healers, mantravadis and magicians. Many of them are not aware that it is an illness. While there are millions of people suffering from various types of mental illnesses, the mental health care facilities available in India are meager.

FACILITIES AVAILABLE IN INDIA

India has made tremendous progress with regard to mental health services in the last two decades.

There are 45 mental hospitals now in India.

The total number of beds now available in these hospitals is around 25,000.

Around 50 percent of these beds are occupied by chronic patients.

Psychiatric departments are functioning in all psychiatric medical colleges in India.

There are a number of private psychiatrists and psychiatric nursing homes available in many parts of the country.

There are around 5000 psychiatrists in India, that is two psychiatrists for one million population, whereas it is 150-200 per million in the developed countries.

Psychiatrists are available in all district hospitals in Tamil Nadu and Kerala.

There are nearly 5000 beds available for psychiatric patients in various general hospitals in India.

Manpower Available (Approximate)

Psychiatrists (qualified)	5000
Clinical psychologists	1000
Psychiatric social workers	2000
Psychiatric nurses	1500
Postgraduate centers in psychiatry	100

Only 10 percent of those requiring active mental health care are receiving the needed help.

In India, there have been a number of innovative approaches to treat and rehabilitate the mentally ill in the last two decades.

The important ones are:

Integrating mental health care with general health care to enable early and regular treatment.

School mental health programs involving the school teachers and students for promotion of mental health as well as care of the ill person.

Promotion of child mental health by the involvement of anganvadis (ICDS programs) and other pre-school child care personnel.

Crisis intervention centers for suicide prevention (Sanjivani Delhi, MPA-Bengaluru, Crisis Intervention Clinic-Government General Hospital, Chennai, Sneha-Chennai, HELF-Mumbai, Saheli-Hyderabad)

Half way homes for the mentally ill for social skills training, vocation training and preparation for community living (Navajeevan-Chennai, MPA and Richmond Fellowship, Bengaluru).

Education of the family of the patient about coping skills, understanding of the illness, supporting in a crisis and reducing family stress and burden (NIMHANS-Bengaluru, Schizophrenia Research Foundation (SCARF) Chennai and other centers at Delhi, Mumbai, Trichy, etc.)

Alcohol and De-addiction centers by Non-Governmental Organizations supported by the Government of India Welfare Department and Voluntary Organizations (e.g. TTR Foundation De-addiction Center-Chennai).

Media materials for public education in the form of books in local language, organizing mental health exhibitions, etc.

Sheltered workshops for the mentally ill and mentally retarded individuals at a number of centers.

NATIONAL MENTAL HEALTH PROGRAM (NMHP)

To create more awareness on mental health among rural people and to give them better mental health care, this community-based mental health program was started in India in 1982. It forms one of the important milestones in Community Psychiatry in India. National Mental Health program was started with the slogan of "Reaching The Unreached". The objectives of National Mental Health Program (NMHP) are:

1. To ensure availability and accessibility of minimum mental health care for all in the foreseeable future, particularly to the most vulnerable and underprivileged section of the population.
2. To encourage affiliation of mental health knowledge in general health care and in social development.
3. To provide community participation in the mental health service development and to stimulate efforts towards self help in the community. NMHP has a phased approach to integrate mental health service with the existing services. It implements its plans by giving short-term training in mental health for PHC medical officer and other paramedical personnel.

DISTRICT MENTAL HEALTH PROGRAM

District Mental Health Program (DMHP) is the basic unit of NMHP.

The DMHP was launched in 1996-1997 in four districts in India one each in AP, TN, Assam, and Rajasthan.

DMHP—The objectives

- To provide sustainable basic mental health services to the community and to integrate these services with other health services
- Early detection. Diagnosis of patients with in the community
- To ensure that patients and their relatives do not have to travel long distances to go to the hospital and nursing homes in cities
- To take pressure off from mental hospitals
- To decrease stigma attached with mental illness through public education and change of attitude
- To treat and rehabilitate patients discharged from the mental hospitals with in the community.

DMHP—Key features

The slates will set in motion the process of finding suitable personnel (mental health team) for manning the DMHP teams. They can take in service candidates and provide them the necessary training in the identified Nodal Institute.

The patients will be from the district itself and adjoining areas.

DMHP will provide service to the needy mentally ill patients and families.

1. Daily OP service.
2. Ten-bedded inpatient service facilities.
3. Referral
4. Liaison with PHCs.
5. Follow-up services.
6. Awareness program.
7. Community surveys (if feasible).

Different times—Different systems:
Custodial care (asylums)
↓
Mental hospitals
↓
Mental health institutes (psychiatric hospital)
Deinstitutionalization
↓
Community care

DMHP is an attempt to decentralize mental health care in the community.

The Essentials of the DMHP are:

1. A decentralized training program for the existing mental health personnel on essentials of mental health care at the district level.
2. Provision of mental health care in all general health facilities.
3. Involvement of all categories of health welfare professionals in mental health care.
4. Provision of psychiatric drugs at all health facilities.
5. A simple record keeping.
6. Mechanisms to monitor the work of PHC personnel in the provision of mental health care.
7. A mental health team at the district level to train personnels.
8. Referral support.
9. Supervision of the MHP.
10. Administrative support of the local Government Health Department.

PROPOSAL FOR 11th 5 YEAR PLAN (2007–2012)

- Expansion of DMHP to 500 districts all over the country with some modifications. Cost of DMHP may be increased to 1.60 crores per district
- A grant of 20 crores has been sought for research purpose. The research areas to be focused included biology of mental diseases, early interventions, improving long-term outcomes in drug/alcohol related disorders
- Improvement in manpower status by:
    a. Increasing number of PG trainees in psychiatry: 50 MD, 25 DPM seats in training colleges
    b. Imparting short-term training courses to GP to train 5000 taluk level medical doctors for 6 months—one year as part of a certified course
- IEC activities: 25 crores budget proposed development of public awareness materials: Posters, radio wordings, video clipping, training mat for UG/PG training: I Interactive CDs
- Support money for implementing MHA and running mental health authorities: (10 crore proposed)
- School Mental Health Program (SMHP): Implemented by imparting life skills education using teachers as trained resource staff
- 100 District. Each year—500.

MENTAL HEALTH SERVICES IN INDIA

WHO Report 2001

The circle of care

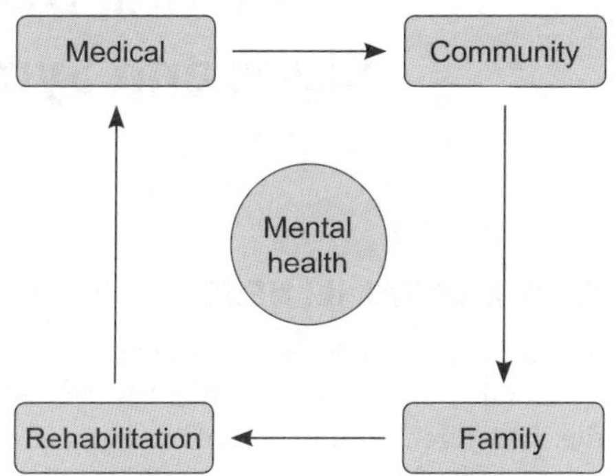

Medical	**Community**
Early recognition	Avoidance of stigma and discrimination
Information about illness and treatment	Full social participation
Medical care	Human rights
Psychological support	
Hospitalization	

Rehabilitation	**Family**
Social support	Skills for care
Education	Family cohesion
Vocational support	Networking with family
Daycare	Crisis support
Long-term care	Financial support
Spiritual needs	Respite care

Chapter

8

Mental Disorders: Signs and Symptoms

THE CONCEPT OF MENTAL ILLNESS

In medical science, the distinction between health and illness or normality and abnormality (literally, 'away from normal') is not difficult to draw. When the integrity; structure and function of an organ or other body part is disturbed or deranged, abnormality exists. In psychological science, however, it is often difficult to distinguish normality from abnormality.

The following models can be used to distinguish normality and abnormality.

Statistical model: The behavior that most people display is considered normal; and behavior that deviates from that of the majority is considered abnormal.

Medical model: Abnormal behavior is 'disease like' and can be diagnosed and treated.

Behavior model: Behavior that is maladaptive is abnormal. Abnormal behavior is a set of a faulty behavior through learning.

Personal distress model: A behavior which is going to produce distress or discomfort to the individual and at times to others is considered to be abnormal.

Legal model: A person's behavior, when he is not able to judge that what he is doing is right or wrong, is abnormal.

But all these models cannot give a satisfying answer to abnormality. Abnormality may differ from culture to culture and country to country. What is considered as abnormal in one culture may be a well accepted norm in another culture.

WHAT IS MENTAL ILLNESS?

In a simple way, it is disorder of the mind. However, it is not so simple so as to describe it in this way.

THE CHARACTERISTICS OF MENTAL ILLNESSES

When a person's behavior is causing distress and suffering to the individual and/or others around him.

Abnormal changes in one's thinking, feeling, memory, perceptions and judgment, resulting in changes in talk and behavior.

Abnormal behavior causes disturbance in the person's day-to-day activities, job and interpersonal relationships.

All the above may be considered as characteristics of mental illness. As somebody put it, "a person who is either sad, bad or odd can be considered abnormal, if these qualities cause problems to him and to others."

THE SIGNS AND SYMPTOMS OF MENTAL ILLNESS

Mental illness can begin suddenly (sudden or acute onset) or emerge slowly over a period of months or even years (insidious onset). If a person suddenly becomes ill, it will be obvious to others that something is wrong. If slow in onset, he may become severely ill before it is discovered. The clinical features may either be very mild or quite severe and obvious to others. Some mentally ill persons will have many of the following signs and symptoms, and some may have only one or two.

General Behavior

Sleep Disturbance

Very common in many mental illnesses. Some patients find it very difficult to get to sleep; others wake during the early hours of the morning and are unable to get back to sleep. Difficulty in getting off to sleep or in maintaining sleep is called Insomnia. Occasionally, some mentally ill people sleep a great deal.

Loss of Appetite and Refusal of Food

This is another common symptom in mental illness. The person who earlier enjoyed food may eat less or never eat at all. This may be due to:

- They may not have any interest in eating because they are depressed, or
- They do not feel hungry, or
- They are too busy to find time to eat (as in Mania), or
- They refuse to eat because they feel that the food is poisoned (as in Paranoid disorder).

Personal Appearance

Personal appearance may be neglected. Some persons are unwilling to shave, take a bath or change their clothes (Schizophrenia); some may dress colorfully (Mania); some may keep their appearance seductive (Hysteria).

Lack of Interest in Sex

Some feel that they have lost their libido. They are not at all interested in their usual sexual activity.

Personal Relationship

They may have strained interpersonal relationship. A person who used to be kind and considerate towards his friends and relatives may become hostile and angry. A friendly person may become withdrawn and aloof. Sometimes, a normally quiet person becomes excited and unnecessarily interferes with others' affairs.

Interest in Work, Hobbies, and Surroundings

May decline; a mentally ill person may give up work because he is no longer interested or unable to do the job. Some patient becomes so dull that they lie in bed all the day.

Behavior

Patients at times behave peculiarly. At times, his behavior irritates others; at times it is dangerous to himself and others. At times, the patient may be overactive and restless and assault others. In contrast, he becomes dull, slow in his activities, refusing to move even to do his personal work (retardation, stupor).

Disturbance in Thinking

Disturbance in thinking can be evident from his talk. At times, the person talks excessively or, in contrast utters only a few words. Some persons may answer, which is in no way related to the question put forth (irrelevant talk). Sometimes, his talk becomes meaningless. There may be no association between sentences or words (incoherent talk).

The train of thought may stop suddenly in the middle of a sentence (thought block). Some patients may have disturbance of thought like thought insertion, though withdrawal, thought broadcasting and thought being controlled by an outside force. These are diagnostic of schizophrenia.

Disorder of the Content of Thought (Delusions)

Delusion is a false fixed belief. It is a disturbance in the content of thinking. The characteristics are:

The person is convinced about a particular belief.

It cannot be corrected by reason or logic.

It is not shared by the members of the same community.

A delusion is primary if it arises on its own and secondary if it is a part of other psychiatric symptoms.

Types of Delusions

Delusions of persecution (paranoid delusion). The person is suspicious of people believes that others are trying to harm him, trying to kill or poison him.

Delusions of grandeur (Grandiose): Suddenly, the person starts to harbor a false belief that he is extraordinarily powerful, wealthy and a very important person. He believes that he can achieve anything and everything, and feels that the entire world is under him.

Delusions of jealousy or infidelity: False belief that his spouse is unfaithful and is having extra-marital affairs.

Delusions of control (Passivity phenomenon): False belief that his thinking, actions and feelings are all not his own but are being controlled by some external agencies.

Nihilistic delusions: The false belief that the world is going to end or his body parts are missing, etc.

Hypochondriacal delusions: False belief that he has some incurable disease.

Delusions can occur in a variety of psychiatric disorders:

In schizophrenia	Paranoid delusions Delusions of control Delusions of infidelity
In mania	Grandiose delusions
In depression	Nihilistic delusions Hypochondriacal delusions
In alcoholism	Delusions of infidelity Persecutory delusions
In organic mental disorders	Persecutory delusions Grandiose delusions

Ideas of Reference

The person has a false idea that people around talk about him and make fun of him.

Obsessional Thought

This is a persistent, recurrent thought, that a person often having, Even though he feels that the thought is absurd, and wants to get rid of it, he cannot do so.

Disturbance of Perception

Illusion

This is a perceptual disturbance, the misinterpretation of a real sensory stimulus.

Example: On seeing a rope in the dark, the person mistakes it for a snake. This can occur in delirium during intoxication.

Hallucination

A hallucination is a false perception which occurs without an external stimulus.

Example: Hearing a voice when no one is around.
Hallucinations can affect any of the five senses.

Auditory hallucination: This is the most common type of hallucination. It is hearing voices when nobody is around. It can occur in schizophrenia, paranoid disorders, and epilepsy and in alcohol withdrawal state.

Visual hallucination: This hallucination consists of seeing figures, objects, shadows, 'ghosts,' etc. When there is actually nothing. Occasionally, it occurs in schizophrenia sign of organic mental disorder, especially epilepsy.

Olfactory hallucination: This hallucination consists smelling pleasant or unpleasant odor in the absence of stimuli. Common in epilepsy (temporal lobe epilepsy).

Gustatory hallucination or hallucination of taste: Usually the person has a peculiar taste in his mouth. This is occasionally present in epilepsy, rarely in paranoid disorder.

Tactile hallucination or hallucination of touch: A feeling of peculiar touch or insects crawling over the body as seen in cocaine intoxication.

Hallucination is usually a sign of mental disorder. Very rarely it can occur in a normal person when he is tired, fatigued or about to fall asleep.

Disturbance of Memory

The ability to remember events can be affected in many psychiatric disorders. Patients suffering from anxiety or depression often complain about forgetting things. It is usually due to lack of interest, agitation or poor registration. Severe memory loss or disturbance can occur in people who are elderly or persons who sustained head injuries.

Amnesia

Amnesia means total loss of memory for a certain period of a person's waking life. The period may vary from a few hours to many months. Amnesia can occur in organic disorders due to brain damage.

Example:

After a head injury

After an attack of epilepsy

After Electroconvulsive therapy.

Amnesia can also occur in functional disorders (non-organic disorders). It may be a result of repression of painful events. At times it may be a sign of hysteria.

Dysmnesia (Paramnesia)

Dysmnesia is the failure of the memory, to recall events that happened minutes or hours ago. It is caused by the damage of the hippocampus and mammillary bodies of the brain. It is a symptom of alcoholic dementia (Korsakoff's psychosis); simplex encephalitis. At times, it may be associated with confabulation (filling up memory gaps with false events).

Organic Memory Impairment

Inability to recall events accurately. Recent events are more difficult to recall than past events. There is poor registration for recent events. This type of memory loss occurs very commonly in dementia.

Consciousness

Consciousness or an awareness of the surroundings become disturbed in some mental illnesses. Apart from unconsciousness, which is a complete loss of awareness, the following conditions are sometimes seen:

Confusion: A confused patient is bewildered by his surroundings. He may find it difficult to express him properly or be able to speak only a few words. Some may wander around not really knowing where they are.

Disorientation: A disoriented patient who is usually very confused may not know the time or place properly or fail to recognize a known person.

Disturbance of Affect or Mood

Mood refers to the internal emotional state of an individual. Affect refers to the external expression of emotional content. A mood state can be considered abnormal if it is inappropriate, deficient or excessive.

The Common Abnormal Mood States

Elation or extreme happiness: Elation is an abnormal mood, it occurs without specific reason. It is a state of marked cheerfulness associated with increased activities, as seen in mania.

Depression: A state of extreme sadness, depression is a symptom of mental illness when it occurs without specific cause, or when it becomes abnormally severe or prolonged. Depression is a state of dejection, hopelessness, sadness and misery.

Anxiety: It is an unpleasant state with anticipation of something harmful. It is a vague fear in the absence of immediate danger. Anxiety is a common experience in everyday life, but in the mentally ill, it can become extremely severe.

Inappropriate affect: When the patient reacts with the wrong emotion to a particular event, for example, a person laughs on hearing about the death of a loved one. It is commonly seen in schizophrenia.

Apathy: This refers to the patient's loss of interest in his surroundings and inability to express feelings. Apathetic patients show little or no emotional response to situations which would arouse normal people. Apathy is a symptom of mental illness, but it can also result from a lack of stimulation in the surroundings.

Incongruous affect: The patient's emotions do not work in harmony with his thoughts, for example, he sheds tears and cries when talking about an amusing event. This is a symptom of schizophrenia.

Disturbance in Motor Activities

Motor behavior sometimes reflects mental functions. Abnormal motor activities peculiar to mental disorders are:

Catalepsy: A general term for immobile position that is constantly maintained.

Waxy flexibility: The person can be 'moulded' into a position which is then maintained. When the examiner moves the person's limb, he feels as if it were made of wax.

Negativism: Motiveless resistance to all attempts to be moved or to all instructions.

Stupor: Lack of reaction to and unawareness of surroundings.

Echopraxia: Pathological imitation of movements of one person by another.

Posturing: Voluntary assumption of bizarre posture and maintaining it for long periods of time.

Chapter

9

Concept of Mental Disorders and Classification

At the outset, we have to understand what abnormality is and who is an abnormal person. In medicine 'abnormality' generally refers to a lack of integrity in any organ, structure or function. The line between normality and abnormality is relatively easy to draw. But in psychiatry, the criteria that divide normal and abnormal behavior are not so easily specified. There are several ways of defining psychological abnormality, and some of these definitions may change from one society to another and from time to time in the same society.

CONCEPT OF ABNORMALITY

A number of criteria have been used to characterize abnormal behavior. The word 'abnormal' means "away from norm".

One definition of abnormality is based on statistical frequency. Abnormal behavior is that is statistically infrequent or deviating from norm.

A person's behavior is considered abnormal when it is not according to the society's standard or expectation.

Abnormal behavior is maladaptive.

A behavior which produces personal distress is considered as abnormal.

As per the Law, a person who is not able to judge what he is doing is right or wrong, is considered abnormal.

Abnormality, as described above, can be assessed by many criteria, but not one is satisfactory. There are various models of psychological disorder.

The medical model: An illness that is caused by a primary etiological agent.

The organic-genetic model: Mental illness is due to the presence of an abnormal gene.

The psychoanalytical model: Mental illness, is due to unconscious conflicts.

Behavioral model: Mental illness is maladjusted behavior, mental symptoms are maladaptive responses.

ETIOLOGY (CAUSES) OF MENTAL DISORDERS

The causes of mental illness are multiple and complex. The causes can be grouped into three major areas.

1. Biological factors
   Genetic (Hereditary)
   Biochemical
   Brain damage
2. Psychological factors—Personality and temperament
   Early upbringing
   Conflicts
3. Social factors
   Loss
   Psychosocial stresses
   Sociocultural factors
   Adversity
   Poverty
   Migration
   Unemployment
   Urbanization.

Biological Factors: Genetic (Hereditary) Factors

In some mental illness, there may be a family member suffering from a similar illness. But in most cases, it is not so. The proneness (risk) for developing mental disorder is transmitted to an individual; but whether the individual would actually manifest the illness depends on many other factors.

Biochemical

Biochemical abnormalities in the brain are considered to be the cause of many psychological disorders. The disturbance in neurotransmitters in the brain is found to play an important role in the etiology of certain psychiatric disorders.

Brain Damage

Any damage to the structure and functioning of the brain can give rise to mental illness. Damage to the structure of the brain may be due to one of the following causes.

- Infection
- Injury
- Intoxication
- Vascular (poor blood supply or bleeding)

- Tumors
- Nutritional
- Degenerative diseases
- Anoxia.

Psychosocial Factors

Personality and temperament may play an important role in the psychosocial make-up of an individual. Each man has his own personality. Personality differs from person to person. It is observed that some specific personality types are more prone to develop certain psychological disorders. For example, those who are a social and reserved (schizoid) are vulnerable to schizophrenia when they face adverse situations and psychosocial stress.

Proper love and affection, suitable guidance and encouragement are necessary for the healthy growth of a person. If they are not available and there are repeated unhappy experiences in childhood that can lead to mental illness in later life.

Frequent quarrels, misunderstanding among family members, lack of warmth and trust among them may adversely influence a person. Such a person, when faced with stress, can break down as he lacks the skills to adjust and control his emotions.

Social Factors

Other factors like poverty, unemployment, injustice, insecurity and severe competitions, migration, urbanization can result in mental distress.

The etiology of mental disorder can be due to the following factors:

Predisposing factors,
Precipitating factors, and
Perpetuating factors.

Predisposing Factors

These make individual susceptible to certain types of mental illness. These are:

Genetic make up
Physical damage to the central nervous system
Adverse psychosocial influence.

Precipitating Factors

Immediate events can trigger off the onset of mental illness. These include:

Physical stress
Psychosocial stress.

Perpetuating Factors

Factors which are responsible for aggravating or prolonging the diseases already existing in an individual.

CLASSIFICATION OF MENTAL DISORDERS

A mental disorder is defined as "a clinically significant behavior or psychological syndrome or pattern that occurs in an individual and that is typically associated with either a painful symptom (distress) or impairment in one or more important areas of functioning (disability)."

A psychiatric disorder can be considered as a disturbance of:
Thought or
cognition or
conation (action or will power) or
Affect (feeling) or
Any imbalance between these factors.

WHY CLASSIFICATION IS NECESSARY

1. A good classification scheme permits reliable diagnosis of individual cases and enables researchers to make studies of the way particular problems develop and the treatment programs that will be most effective.
2. Classification of mental disorders is essential as it provides a better way of communicating with others. Also, it gives clear guidelines for a diagnosis, which is reliable and valid.
3. Classification also helps in better management.
4. Classification gives clues for predicting the outcome of mental disorder.

At present, there are two major internationally accepted classifications available in psychiatry.

ICD-10: International Classification of Mental and Behavioral disorders by World Health Organization (WHO).

DSM- V: Diagnostic and Statistical Manual of Mental Disorders by American Psychiatric Association (APA), officially practiced in India

- The major groups of mental disorders as found in ICD-10 are
- Organic, including symptomatic mental disorders
- Mental and behavioral disorders due to psychoactive substance abuse
- Schizophrenia, schizotypal and delusional disorders
- Mood (affective) disorders
- Neurotic, stress-related and somatoform disorders
- Behavioral syndromes associated with physiological disturbances and physical factors

- Disorders of adult personality and behavior
- Mental retardation
- Disorders of psychological development
- Behavioral and emotional disorders with onset usually in childhood and adolescence
- Unspecified mental disorder.

However, for the purpose of this book, **a simple, but practical classification** is adapted as follows:

1. Organic mental disorders
   Delirium (Acute organic mental disorder)
   Dementia (Chronic organic mental disorder)
2. Functional (non-organic) mental disorders
   A. Psychotic disorders
      Schizophrenia
      Mood (affective) disorder
      Delusional (paranoid) disorder
   B. Neurotic disorders
      Anxiety disorders (Generalized anxiety disorder, panic disorder and phobic disorder)
      Obsessive compulsive disorder.
3. Personality disorders.
4. Psychosexual disorders.
5. Stress-related disorders
   Acute stress reaction
   Posraumatic stress disorder
   Adjustment disorder.
7. Mental disorders due to psychoactive substance abuse
   A. Alcohol dependence
   B. Other drugs dependence
   C. Somatoform disorders
      Dissociative (Conversion disorder)
      - Hysteria
      - Hypochondriasis
      - Somatization disorder.
8. Psychosomatic (psychophysiological) disorders.
9. Child psychiatric disorders
   Autism
   Developmental disorders
   Mental retardation
   Attention deficit disorders
   Conduct disorders

Emotional disorders
Habit disorders

10. Other disorders
    Eating disorders
    Disorders of sleep
    Disorders of memory
    Epilepsy and psychiatric aspects
    Psychiatric disturbances in women
    Psychiatric disturbances in adolescents
    Psychiatric disturbances in old age.

Chapter 10

Psychiatric Examination

Psychiatric examination consists mainly of interviews with patient and with his close relatives, if necessary.

FORMAT FOR EXAMINING PSYCHIATRIC PATIENTS

Basic Information

Name:
Age:
Sex:
Occupation:
Address:

Complaints

Patient's main problem is symptoms and abnormal behavior. If the patient is unable to tell psychiatric history, get it from a close relative.

History of Present Illness

Onset:
Precipitating factors:
Course:

Previous Illnesses

Psychiatric:
Physical:

Personal Life History

Birth:
Childhood:
Education:

Occupation:
Marriage:
Sexual practices:
Menstrual history (female patients):
Habits, like alcohol, drugs and smoking:
Religious practices, hobbies, interests:
Daily activity:

Family History

Family background:
Parents and siblings:
Family history of mental illness:

Personality

What type of person is he or she:
Reserved (introvert):
Social (extrovert):
Suspicious (paranoid):
Perfectionist (obsessive):
Hysterical:
Antisocial:
Aggressive:
Frequent mood changes (cyclothymic):

Mental Status Examination

Appearance, Attitude and Behavior

General description:
Behavior and psychomotor activity:
Attitude towards examiner:

Speech

Relevant/irrelevant:
Coherent/incoherent:

Mood (Affect) and Emotion State

Subjective feeling:
The interviewer's observation:
Appropriateness:

Thought Process and Content

Production of thought:
Continuity of thought:
Content of thought:
Preoccupation with suicidal ideas:
Delusion:

Perception

Illusion:
Hallucination:

Attention and Concentration

Days of week backwards, months of year backward, serial subtraction of seven from hundred:

Orientation

Time (day, date):
Place:
Person:

Memory

Immediate: Give an address and ask him to repeat after five minutes.
Recent: What he has taken for breakfast in the morning. Experience in the last few days, TV, radio news, etc.
Remote: Past personal events like school, marriage.

Intelligence

Simple arithmetic calculation:
General knowledge:
Reading, writing:

Abstract Thinking

Proverb testing (The moral behind the proverb).

Judgment

What would you do if a nearby hut is on fire?
What would you do if you found a stamped addressed letter on the road?

Insight

Whether the person knows that he is mentally ill or not and to what extent?

The Role of a Nurse in Writing a Relevant Case Sheet

The nurse should write the case record clearly and precisely. She should avoid lengthy notes.

As much as possible, use special and technical terminology, e.g. the person has grandiose delusion with auditory hallucination.

Use the patient's own words and quote whenever possible when describing an important sign.

Give specific examples instead of your own interpretations, e.g. do not write 'patient was angry' But write, "Patient dashed out of the door and shouted at me."

Sign the note, so that the reader knows who is making the observation.

Chapter

11

Anxiety Disorders (Neurotic Disorders)

Neurosis (plural-neuroses) is a less severe form of psychological disorder where patients show either excessive or prolonged emotional reaction to any given stress. They have symptoms like anxiety, fear, sadness, vague aches and pains and other bodily symptoms. They are aware of their problems and seek help.

The basic and predominant features of anxiety disorders are tension, fear or worry. All people get tensed or worried from time-to-time especially when faced with difficult problems, however, they are able to cope with the situations and overcome these tensions. If the tension is too intense or prolonged in duration, they tend to interfere with the person's sense of well-being and disturb his normal functioning. The primary symptom of neurosis is anxiety.

In traditional usage, neurosis is a psychological disturbance in which there are one or more symptoms, such as phobia, obsession or compulsion that are ineffective attempts to deal with anxiety. There are no clear-cut organic brain related problems, no violation of basic social norms, no loss of orientation to reality, but the individual still shows a life-long pattern of self-defeating and inadequate coping strategies aimed at reducing anxiety.

CHARACTERISTICS OF NEUROTIC PERSONS

There is no clear line between neurotic and normal individuals.

The difference between the two is only depend upon their minor behavioral changes.

Many neurotics basically have feelings of inadequacy and inferiority (lack of confidence) which lead them to see their day-to-day problems as difficult and threatening.

The neurotic is constantly under tension and worry, and has multiple, vague bodily complaints.

Neurotic people are inclined to be more sensitive, more emotional and less reliable than normal individuals,

Neurotics rely greatly upon other people, are often possessive and seldom independent. Frequently, they are insecure people.

They may seek to protect themselves emotionally and therefore often appear selfish.

Because of their personality traits, neurotic people frequently experience difficulties in their relationship with colleagues, friends and relatives. Difficult personal relationships only worsen the matters and produce further problems.

Neurotic behavior patterns vary considerably, though all share a common mechanism for limiting anxiety.

The neurotic lives a life in which he or she see 'no exit' from life's problems and no choices among different ways of being.

They are confined in a psychological prison in which the mind is both jailer and the prisoner.

CAUSES OF NEUROSIS (ANXIETY DISORDERS)

Freud was the first to point out that neurosis is caused by mental conflicts. Causes of neurosis are manifold. They are:

Intrapsychic Conflict (Conflict Within the Mind)

This conflict is unconscious and not readily understood by the patient. However, it causes tremendous amount of anxiety and related problems. Sexual conflict can also produce neurosis.

Interpersonal Problems

This includes problems in the family, at work or with friends.

The Environmental Stress

This includes loss of loved one, failure, disappointment and frustrations. A severe stress can precipitate neurosis even in a stable personality.

The Individual Susceptibility

This depends upon the personality make-up of the individual and also early-life experience.

Freud termed nearly all forms of behavior associated with anxiety as neuroses. Freud's term, neurosis has made its way into everyday language and common people tend to describe any behavioral abnormality as neurotic. Now, it is believed by many psychiatrists that the term neurosis is not always appropriate.

Nearly 10 percent of the population suffers from neurosis. (Anxiety disorders) Neurosis forms 30 percent of the general practitioners' cases and nearly 60 percent of the Psychiatrists' practice.

Neurotic	Psychotic
The neurotic frequently talks about his symptoms	The psychotic often denies that there is anything wrong with him (lack of insight)
The neurotic does not lose contact with reality	The psychotic loses contact with reality
Personality is intact	Personality is often disorganized and deteriorates
Neurotics continue to function socially and at work	Psychotics cannot act normally in society and may harm himself or others
Hospitalization is not usually required	Often requires hospitalization

As per some new classification of mental disorders, most of the disorders formerly covered in a category called neurosis are delineated into anxiety, somatoform and dissociative disorders.

Common Neurotic Disorders (Anxiety Disorder)

Anxiety disorder
Generalized anxiety disorder
Panic disorder
Phobic disorder
Obsessive compulsive disorder
Hysterical disorder → Somatoform disorders
Hypochondriacal disorder → Somatoform disorders

Anxiety Disorders

Anxiety is a common emotion in everyone's experience. It is a universal human experience. W.H. Auden called the modern era as the" Age of Anxiety". The current conflicts in civilization leads to urbanization and industrialization and the rapid changes in our environment, all pave way for more anxiety prone situations. Anxiety occupies a central position in our psychic apparatus or mind. Anxiety is one of the central factors in both normal and abnormal behavior.

Anxiety is a motivating force to an intrapsychic urge and a certain minimum level of anxiety improves performances in many situations.

Thus, anxiety is considered as a normal experience. Anxiety is a common symptom in all forms of emotional illnesses. When it is intense and severe, and when it disturbs the internal psychological equilibrium, we call anxiety as abnormal. Anxiety is also a symptom in many physical illnesses. Anxiety itself forms a separate disorder on its own right. Thus,

Anxiety is a normal experience.

It is symptom of many psychological and physical disorders, and

It is a disorder of its own.

Anxiety is an unpleasant emotion, so that many who experience it, urgently seek relief. Anxiety is the base for most of the stress related and psychosomatic disorders.

Anxiety is the basic symptom of many neurotic disorders. Anxiety disorders are psychological disturbances where anxiety is the essential symptom. Anxiety disorders are classified into:

Generalized anxiety disorder

Panic disorder

Phobic disorder

Obsessive compulsive disorder

Generalized Anxiety Disorder (GAD)

Generalized anxiety disorder is characterized by a generalized, persistent anxiety of at least six months duration, and manifested by Signs of motor tension, autonomic hyperactivity, apprehensive expectation and vigilance.

Generalized anxiety disorder is the most common neurotic disorder. It occurs more frequently in women. Life-time prevalence is estimated as 3–17 per 1000 among men, and 1 – 38 per 1000 among women. Not everyone with anxiety seeks medical help.

This long-term anxiety is called Free Floating Anxiety if it has no obvious source.

The symptoms of GAD vary from individual to individual. The patients do not report acute fluctuation in their anxiety level. They experience persistent and diffuse anxiety. Generalized anxiety; disorder manifests with both physical and psychological signs and symptoms.

Physical Symptoms of GAD

Cardiovascular system

Tachycardia

Chest pain

Palpitations

Dropped beats

Flushing

Fainting

Respiratory system
Sighing
Choking
Yawning
Dyspnea

Alimentary system
Dry mouth
Dysphagia
Dyspepsia
'Butterflies' in stomach
Nausea
Abdominal pain
Diarrhea

Genitourinary system
Frequency
Hesitation
Sexual dysfunction

Nervous system
Tension headaches
Blurring of vision
Tinnitus
Sweating
Tremor
Dilated pupils

Musculoskeletal system
Aches and pain
Teeth clenching
Chronic jerks.

Psychological Symptoms of Anxiety
Anxious mood (Feeling of something terrible about to happen)
Worry or fear
Irritability
Inability to relax
Feeling of being unable to cope
Feeling restless
Depersonalization
Derealization
Initial insomnia
Nightmares.

Panic Disorder

Panic disorder is defined as a sudden attack of intense discomfort, fear or terror. Panic disorder is characterized by fear and subsequent attempts to avoid of specific objects or situations, which the person thinks are unreasonable. Panic disorder is a powerful event. Panic attack with its psychological and somatic symptoms is seen as a horrifying and threatening experience. Attacks usually occur without warning. They may occur as isolated events, and in patients with depression and anxiety disorder. Often panic disorders are seen at the casualty, or as an emergency in a consulting room.

Psychological Symptoms of Panic Disorder

Intense anxiety

Fear of dying or losing control

Depersonalization

Derealization.

Physical Symptoms of Panic Disorder

Increased heart rate

Dizziness

Sweating

Trembling

Dyspnea

Gastrointestinal disorders and others.

Etiology of GAD and Panic Disorders

Generalized anxiety disorders is more frequent among relatives of patients with this condition.

Biochemical disturbance in neurotransmitters especially noradrenalin, serotonin and GABA may cause anxiety disorder.

Psychological as a result of intrapsychic conflict, as a conditioned response—(maladaptive learning).

Management of GAD and Panic Disorder

Includes:

Evaluation of the patient's symptoms.

Detailed history.

Understanding the relationship between symptoms and life events.

Determination of a treatment plan.

Drug Treatment in Anxiety Disorders

Benzodiazepines—Diazepam	5-15 mg per day
Chlordiazepoxide	10-30 mg per day
Clonazepam	0.5-2 mg
Alprazolam	0.5-3 mg per day (the drug of choice in panic attack)
Lorazepam	1-3 mg per day
Flurazepam	10-30 mg per day
Buspirone	10-30 mg per day
Beta-blockers—Propranolol	20-120 mg per day (more useful in reducing physical symptoms).

Psychological Methods of Treatment

Explanation
Reassurance
Crisis intervention
Supportive psychotherapy
Relaxation exercises
Group therapy
Yoga and meditation.

Phobic Disorder

A phobia is an unreasonable fear of an object or situation. The phobia patient will be terrified when confronted with these situations and the symptoms will be similar to those of an acute attack of anxiety.

Fear is a rational reaction to an object, identified external danger (such as fire in one's home or seeing a snake inside the house) and may involve flight or attack in self defense. In contrast, a person with a phobic disorder recognizes that he or she is suffering from a persistent and irrational fear of some specific object, activity, or situation (the phobic stimulus) that causes a compelling desire to avoid it (the phobic reaction).

Phobias are divided into three groups:
Simple phobia,
Agoraphobia,
Social phobia. (Social anxiety disorders).

The phobia becomes a neurosis if it incapacitates the patient. Most of the cases that seek psychiatric treatments are of agoraphobia.

Simple Phobia (Specific Phobia)

A disorder characterized by irrational and persistent fear of an object or situation, along with a compelling desire to avoid it. Usually, it is the fear of harmless animals or objects and certain situations like, fear of insects, small animals, height, dark places, examinations, closed spaces, sight of blood, marriage, travel, etc.

Fear of closed spaces	Claustrophobia
Fear of the sight of blood	Hematophobia
Fear of height	Acrophobia
Fear of marriage	Gamophobia
Fear of insects	Insectophobia
Fear of cats	Ailurophobe
Fear of dogs	Cynophobia
Fear of dirt	Mysophobia
Fear of darkness	Nyctophobia
Fear of death	Thanatophobia
Fear of AIDS	AIDS phobia
Fear of venereal diseases	Venereophobia

Agoraphobia

A disorder characterized by fear of being alone in an open space (public place) and in crowds from which escape might be difficult. This condition is more incapacitating because it restricts the patient's daily activities. The fear can become debilitating, and some individuals avoid going into any open space, traveling in aeroplanes or being in a crowd. People with severe cases may decide never to leave their homes. Agoraphobia is often precipitated by stress, particularly interpersonal stress. It is far more common in women than in men.

Social Phobia

A disorder characterized by fear of and desire to avoid situation in which the person might be exposed to scrutiny by others and might behave in an embarrassing or humiliating way. This is a fear of appearing shameful or stupid or of blushing in the presence of others.

Treatment of Phobic Disorders

Drug Treatment: Antianxiety drugs like diazepam, chlordiazepoxide, clonazepam, alprazolam and propranolol should be used as a short-term treatment.

Behavior therapy: Long-term treatment consists of behavioral therapy. This includes:

Systematic desensitization: The patient is exposed gradually to the situations or objects of his or her phobia.

Flooding: Sudden exposure of the patient to the phobic situation until he is no more fearful.

Implosion: Flooding technique carried out in imagination.

Obsessive Compulsive Disorder (OCD)

This disorder is characterized by persistent and uncontrollable thoughts and irrational beliefs that cause an individual to perform compulsive rituals that interferes with his or her daily life. Patients have either recurrent, persistent ideas, thoughts or images (obsessions), or repetitive, stereotyped, seemingly purposeless behavior (compulsions).

Even though the person feels that the thoughts are absurd and wants to avoid them, they will keep coming with more and more force. They produce a lot of anxiety which the patient has difficulty in controlling. The important categories of obsessions are:

Dirt and contamination
Aggression
Orderliness
Sex
Religion.

A compulsion is a repetitive act carried out in a stereotyped manner. It may manifest itself as repeated washing of hands; a long time over baths, repeated checking or counting, setting in order or arranging compulsive urge to tell or ask something or confess.

Obsessions and compulsions may occur separately, but they are together so often that they are considered two aspects of a single disorder.

There is always an accompanying anxiety that leads one with the OCD to take counter measures against certain ideas or impulses. The obsession or compulsion is not a casual part of one's self. It is undesired, unacceptable and uncontrollable. The idea or the impulse is intrusive and unwanted originating from within the person's own mind and is recognized as senseless, absurd or irrational accompanied with a strong feeling to resist them.

OCD is of gradual onset. The illness usually lasts for an year or more before the patient seeks consultation. OCD is very common and about one to three percent of the general population suffers from it. It is more common in younger age groups in both sexes.

Causes of OCD

The exact cause is not known. However, the biochemical cause is more widely accepted nowadays. It is believed that deficiency of serotonin, a neurotransmitter, probably plays an important role in causing OCD. Hereditary factors, a morbid, obsessive personality, upbringing, (Anankastic personality) childhood experiences, intrapsychic conflicts. All are considered to have some role in the etiology of OCD.

Treatment of OCD

Drug Treatment

The antidepressant clom ipramine is considered to be an effective drug in managing OCD. Fluoxetine, another antidepressant is also considered to be effective (20–120 mg/day). Sertralin, fluvoxamine and paroxetine are other useful drugs.

Psychological Methods of Treatment

Supportive Psychotherapy

Behavior therapy

(Desensitization and flooding—for obsessional fears
Thought stopping—for obsessional thoughts
Exposure and response prevention—for compulsive behavior).
Cognitive behavior therapy (CBT).

Nursing Care In OCD

Therapeutic Needs

Physical Needs

- Encourage personal hygiene
- Care of skin
- Improve appetite and weight
- Improve sleep pattern.

Psychosocial Needs

Psychotherapeutic environment
Help in coping with obessive compulsive behavior
Improving communication
Enhance self concept and socialization
Reduce anxiety.

Recreational Activities

Playing games
Hearing music
Exercise
Dancing

Spiritual Needs

Meditation
Yoga
Moral Stories.

Discharge Plan

Follow-up care
Health education.

HYSTERIA

Hysteria is a common type of neurosis. Hysteria continues to be a common clinical problem in psychiatric and non-psychiatric medical practice.

Contrary to reports from the West, there is no evidence to suggest a decline in the number of hysterical patients in our country.

About two percent of our population suffers from hysteria. Hysteria is more common in women than in men. It is commoner in young women and adolescent girls.

Patients with hysteria have multiple vague bodily complaints which mimic neurological or physical disorders. Physical examination does not reveal any abnormality and investigations are negative.

The Multiple Meaning of Hysteria

Several authors have emphasized the multiple meanings attached to the term hysteria:

Hysterical personality.
Conversion hysteria.
Dissociative states.
St Louis hysteria (Briquet's syndrome).
Epidemic hysteria (Mass hysteria).

Common Characteristics of Hysteria

They correspond to an idea in the mind of the patient concerning physical or sensory changes or psychological function.

They are definable as somatic in terms of positive evidence as psychological by clinical examinations.

They are related to emotional conflict—a patient develops hysterical symptom when she faces stress intolerable.

Primary gain—reduction of anxiety.
Secondary gain—advantages, sympathy, or concession.
Symbolic choice of symptom.
Manipulation of other persons and the environment.
Hysterical personality.

Hysterical Personality (Histrionic personality)

An hysterical personality is immature, dependent, possessive, seductive but frigid. She is demanding, manipulate, overt demonstrative and has a tendency to pretend, tell fantastic lies and behave in a dramatic way. She is unreliable and attention seeking, craving for appreciation, is flamboyant and exhibitionistic and suggestible.

Conversion Hysteria (Conversion disorder)

This is defined as the subconscious process through which anxiety is converted into physical symptoms. Thus, an emotional conflict is converted into a physical problem.

Conversion symptoms are expressed in many ways. These principally occur as disorders of mobility or perception.

- Hysterical seizures (Fits)
- Hysterical paralysis
- Hysterical blindness
- Hysterical aphonia
- Hysterical anesthesia
- Psychogenic pain.

Conversion disorders are associated with increased stress, repressed ideas and maladaptive coping methods. Conversion disorders have no organic cause. There will be labelle indifference, for example; the blind person is not concerned about blindness when she describes her loss of sight. The symptoms appear in sudden and dramatic manner and often arouse lot of anxiety in the patient's relatives.

Dissociative Disorder

This is an anxiety-relieving, hysterical problem. Here, the person dissociates or separates himself from the original self and acts in a new manner.

The common manifestations are:
Hysterical amnesia and fugue states.
Hysterical trance states (possession syndrome).
Multiple personality.

Hysterical Amnesia

The patient has loss of memory, which may cover a period of days or weeks to years. There is a sudden inability to recall important personal information. The extent of the disturbance is too great to be explained by ordinary forgetfulness. The amnesia may be localized, generalized, selective or continuing in nature.

Fugue

Fugue (Wandering in a dazed state). It could be manifested as a sudden unexpected journey from home or work location with the assumption of a new identity and an inability to recall the past. Following recovery, there is no recollection of events that took place during the fugue. The course is typically brief, hours to days and rarely months.

Hysterical Trance

A trance is a ritualistic dance-like behavior usually performed during religious ceremonies. The person in a trance state may feel that a spirit has entered her body and believe that she has the power to heal the sick, communicate with the dead or to predict the future.

Hysterical Possession State

It is a hysterical tans state. A culture-bound syndrome, which is very common in our country.

Especially in South, the patient, usually a female, behaves as if she is possessed by a god or goddess. It is well accepted that some individuals use this symptom to express their inner conflicts and get a solution in a socially accepted manner. Majority of them are treated by traditional healers like priests, faith healers, mantravadis and fakirs. Only a small percent of them seek medical or psychiatric help. Except during the possession state, the individual remains apparently normal. Hindus believe in possession traditionally. The person is not blamed for his abnormal behavior and gets attention; she also gets a socially recognized status of being possessed. A definite psychological precipitating factor is found in majority of the cases.

Multiple personality: The existence within the individual of two or more distinct personalities one of which is dominant at a particular time. The original personality usually is not aware (at least initially) of the existence of such personalities. Transition from one personality to another is sudden and often associated with psychological stress. The course tends to be more chronic.

Management of Hysteria

The main aim is to restore the lost function gradually rather than suddenly. A careful history and a thorough understanding of the personality of the patient is the basic step of management of hysteria.

Psychological Methods of Treatment

Psychotherapy including suggestion, explanation, persuasion and encouragement.

Psychoanalytic psychotherapy, if the problem is intense and deep-rooted.

Hypnotherapy.

Physical Method of Treatment

Abreaction or pentothol analysis to understand the inner conflict and to remove the symptoms.

Antianxiety and antidepressant drugs for a short-term period may be beneficial.

HYPOCHONDRIASIS

Hypochondrial patients are characteristically anxious and too much concerned about their health. They are preoccupied with the functioning of their bodies. Despite repetitive assurance that there is no major disease, the patient still feels that some underlying disease has not been diagnosed; believes that he has some incurable disease.

The symptoms are different and involving many different areas of the body. The common sites are abdomen, chest, head and neck. In fact, the symptoms may be related to any part of the body or the general, like fatigue. The patients go from doctor to doctor undergoing endless examinations and investigations, in turn picking up many medical terms and suffering from more anxiety and more hypochondriasis.

Nowadays, the term somatization disorder is replacing 'hypochondriasis. Somatization disorder is characterized by recurrent and multiple complaints of long duration for which medical attention has been ineffective.

Somatization is expressing their psychological problem through bodily symptoms since in our country, people give more attention to somatic symptoms than psychological problems.

NURSING CARE OF ANXIETY DISORDER

Explain to the patient and relatives that the symptoms are not due to any physical disease but due to a mild psychological problem which can be effectively treated.

Reassure the patient that many people have similar problems, it is short lived and can be managed effectively.

Be supportive to the patient and to the relatives.

Patient develops a feeling of security in the presence of a calm and tactful nurse.

Patients suffering from panic disorders may fear for his or her life, and need support and reassurance.

Keep the surrounding low in stimuli (dim lighting, few people). A stimulating environment may increase the level of anxiety.

The nurse should identify the precipitating factor and educate the patient to avoid it.

Help the patient understand the benefit of relaxation in anxiety-provoking situation and teach them simple relaxation techniques, deep-breathing exercises, physical exercise like a brisk walk, jogging, meditation and so on. A relaxed body will help to relax the mind.

It is important for a nurse to understand the patient's fear and help him or her to reduce it.

The nurse should educate the patient to accept the reality.

The nurse should understand the ineffective coping in anxiety disorder and teach the patient better coping strategies.

Especially in OCD, positive reinforcement enhances self-esteem and encourages repetition of desired behavior. Anxiety is minimized when the patient is able to replace ritualistic behavior with more adaptive ones.

It is essential for the nursing care to encourage patients with anxiety disorder to take care of their own activities without much assistance.

Patient's comfort and safety are nursing priorities.

The nurse dealing with an anxiety disorder patient should be careful in not allowing the patient become dependent on the nursing staff.

Too much dependence will interfere with the therapeutic relationship.

Abreaction (pentothal analysis)

Hypnosis

Psychotherapy.

NURSING CARE IN ANXIETY DISORDERS

Therapeutic Needs

Effective nurse-relationship

Abreaction

Hypnosis

Psychotherapy.

Physical Needs

Improve sleep pattern

Decreased activity, restlessness

Improve hydration

Improve appetite and weight.

Psychosocial Needs

Decreased activity
Improve perception, communication, coping abilities, socialization, and family support.

Recreational Activities

Playing games
Hearing music
Exercise
Dancing.

Spiritual Needs

Meditation
Yoga
Moral Stories.

Discharge Plan

Follow-up care
Health education.

Nursing Care in Hysteria

The nurse should identify the problem and reassure the relatives that it can be controlled and that there is no organic base for the symptom. However, it is not advisable to tell the relatives that she is acting or malingering. Rather, one must say that it is a subconscious emotional problem, which is to be attended.

To the patient the nurse should be a sympathetic listener and must never tell the patient that she has no problem. The nurse should give an impression to the patient that her problem could be resolved.

The nurse should give an impression to the patient that she is very concerned, thereby establishing a rapport and gaining the patient's confidence.

What the patient actually needs is attention and sympathy. If she can ventilate her feelings, most of the problem will be solved.

Nurse should give reassurance, support and insight-oriented psychotherapy.

Before starting the therapeutic approach the patient's personality has to be fully assessed and her cultural background should be understood by the nurse.

Identification of the precipitating stressor is important for assessment purposes. This will be useful in helping the patient to cope more adaptively.

Patient's comfort and safety are nursing priorities.

Allow the patient to express her feelings and emotional conflicts.

Establish trusting relationship with patient. Trust enhances therapeutic interactions between nurse and patient.

Identify the gains that the physical symptoms have provided for the patient.

Do not focus on disability and allow patient to be as independent as possible. Nurse should intervene only when patient requires assistance. Allow and encourage the patient to perform normal activities. Encourage independence. Take care not to foster dependency.

Remember that the physical symptoms are real to the patient; it is not in the patient's conscious control.

NURSING PROCESS IN HYSTERIA

Therapeutic Needs

Physical Needs

Enhance self-esteem
Improve communication
Improve socialization
Decreased concern of physical symptoms and self-centered speech.

Psychosocial Needs

Decreased attention—seeking mechanism
Appropriate use of emotions
Decreased maladaptive behavior
Decreased manipulative behavior.

Recreational Needs

Art, music, dance, and sports.

Spiritual Needs

Prayer, yoga, and meditation.

Discharge Plan

Follow-up care.

Nursing Care in Dissociative Disorder

The nurse's presence must reassure the patient as dissociative behavior is frightening to the patient.

Do not flood the patient with data regarding his or her past life. Individuals who are exposed to painful information from which the amnesia is providing protection may relapse.

Expose patient to stimuli that represents pleasant experiences to the patient. As memory begins to return, engage patient in activities. Patient to discuss situations that have been especially stressful, and to explore the feelings associated with those times. Identify conflicts and help the patient find possible solutions.

Chapter

12

Adjustment Disorders

An **adjustment disorder** is a maladaptive reaction to a clearly identifiable psychosocial stressor or stressors that occur within three months after the stressor's onset. It is a pathological response to a personal misfortune. Adjustment disorder is a new name for describing a mild maladaptive reaction to a clearly identifiable adverse event. Adjustment disorder can be considered to be the common cold of psychiatry. Duration of the symptoms is less than 6 months.

SUBTYPES OF ADJUSTMENT DISORDERS

- Adjustment disorder with depressed mood: Major symptoms include depressed mood, tearfulness and hopelessness
- Adjustment disorder with anxious mood: The major symptoms include nervousness, worry and jitteriness.
- Adjustment disorder with mixed emotions: Symptoms of both depression and anxiety disorders are present.
- Adjustment disorders with disturbance of conduct: Symptoms of conduct disorder, like violation of the rights of others or social norms.
- Adjustment disorder with mixed disturbance of emotions and conduct: Manifestations are both emotional (depression, anxiety) and disturbances in conduct.
- Adjustment disorder with work or academic institution: Impairment of occupation ability and academic performance.
- Adjustment disorder with withdrawal: The predominant manifestation is social withdrawal.
- Adjustment disorder with physical complaints: The manifestation involves physical symptoms such as headache, backache and other vague complaints.

ETIOLOGY

Faulty rearing habit—It is the mother's inability to allow the child to become independent, which leads to problems with adjustment in later life.

The individual is unable to successfully complete age-appropriate tasks. There is often retarded ego development and the inability to use ego defense mechanisms appropriately.

Persons with adjustment difficulties experience negative learning. There is inadequate role model in family system. The disturbed family pattern damages the self-esteem, which also contributes to maladaptive adjustment responses.

TREATMENT OPTIONS IN ORDER OF PREFERENCE

Brief psychotherapy
Short-term course of antianxiety drugs
Long-term individual psychodynamic psychotherapy
Group psychotherapy
Observation.

NURSING CARE FOR PERSONS WITH ADJUSTMENT DISORDERS

The nurse should basically understand that the person suffers from stress and his response to the stress is maladaptive. It is maladaptive because there is an impairment in social or occupational functioning. The behaviors are exaggerated. Hence, the basic task of the nurse is to teach and train the person to effectively cope with his stress in the usual manner.

This requires:

Careful observation of the patient's behavior.

Observing for any suicidal behavior or expression.

Providing an opportunity to vent his feelings and assure him with positive goals.

Reassurance and supportive psychotherapy does a lot of good.

Channelizing the anger and violent behavior into physical exercise (e.g. walking, jogging, playing games). Physical exercise is a safe and effective way of relieving pent-up tension.

Listen and talk to the patient frequently.

Maintain a common attitude to patient.

Administer tranquilizing drugs as advised by the doctor.

Do not debate, argue, rationalize or bargain with the patient.

Chapter 13

Personality Disorders

Personality can be defined as the sum total of a person's intellectual, emotional and volitional traits; and it is revealed by his appearance, behavior, habits and relationship with other people, which differentiate him as unique individual.

Personality disorder is defined as the possession of one or more personality traits so deviated from the normal that they interfere with his well-being or adjustment to society and require psychiatric attention.

CHARACTERISTICS OF PERSONALITY DISORDER

It is not a mental illness:

- It is a maladaptive behavior
- It is the possession of abnormal personality traits
- It is a long lasting, most of the time life-long problem
- It causes significant impairment in social or occupational functioning
- It produces distress to the individual and to others.

Personality disorder is different from mental illness. The symptoms of mental illness are mostly episodic and not continuous, whereas the symptoms of personality disorders are continuous and start from adolescence or even before. These patients are odd but not mad.

Personality disorder increases vulnerability to mental illness and also worsens the course and treatment response, especially in depression, anxiety and drug and alcohol abuse.

About ten percent of the outpatient psychiatric population and five percent of the inpatient psychiatric population may be diagnosed as suffering from personality disorders. It is most commonly found in the age group of 18–35 years and in more common in males and lower social classes.

Personality disorders can be classified into four groups.

Withdrawn (odd and eccentric)

Schizotypal
Schizoid
Paranoid.

Dependent (anxious and fearful)

Anxious (avoidant)
Dependent
Passive aggressive.

Inhibited

Anankastic (obsessive compulsive)
Hypochondriacal
Depressive (Dysthymic).

Antisocial (Dramatic, emotional, flamboyant and erratic)

Histrionic
Impulsive co-borderline
Narcissistic
Psychopathic.

MAIN PERSONALITY DISORDERS

Paranoid personality disorder: Oversensitivity, tendency to bear grudges, suspiciousness, misconstruing neutral or friendly actions of others.

Schizoid personality disorder: Emotional coldness, preference for fantasy, introspective, reserved, little interest in having sexual experiences with others, lack of close and confiding relationships.

Anxious (avoidant) personality disorder: Pervasive tension and apprehension, self-consciousness, hypersensitivity to rejection, entering into relationships only if guaranteed uncritical acceptance, exaggerating potential dangers and risks in everyday situations and avoiding certain activities, leading to a restricted lifestyle .

Dependent personality disorder: Encourages or allows others to assume responsibility for major areas of the individual's life; subordinate to, complaint about and unwilling to make demands on those on whom they depend. Perceives self as helpless, fears of being abandoned and left alone, devastated when close relationships end.

Anankastic (obsessive-compulsive) personality disorder: Indecisiveness, perfectionism, excessive conscientiousness, pedantry and conventionality, rigidity and stubbornness, planning all activities far ahead in minute detail.

Histrionic personality disorder: Dramatic, overemotional, suggestible, shallow and labile effectivity, craves attention, and manipulative.

Emotionally unstable impulsive type personality disorder: Emotionally unstable, lack of impulse control, outbursts of violence or threatening behavior.

Borderline type personality disorder: Unclean or disturbed self-image, intense and unstable relationships, which may lead to repeated emotional crises that may be associated with a series of suicidal threats or acts of self-harm.

Psychopathic (antisocial) personality disorder: Abnormally aggressive and extremely irresponsible person whose behavior brings him repeatedly into conflict with society and the law.

Its prevalence varies from 0.06 percent to 1.5 percent. The person usually comes from a deprived or broken family, or having an alcoholic or psychopathic parent.

CLINICAL FEATURES OF PSYCHOPATHIC PERSONALITY DISORDERS

The patient is basically a guiltless and loveless individual, highly impulsive in nature, with no regret for his misdeeds. He lacks normal drive or motivation. He cannot establish a sustained relationship with anybody. Superficially charming but can quickly becomes irritable and highly selfish. He has low frustration tolerance and blames others for his behavior. He does not learn from his experiences, so again and again commits the same mistakes or criminal behavior.

There is usually a history of stealing, lying, fighting, running away from home and cruelty to animals from childhood to adolescence which continues in adult life. He may cheat, misappropriate funds, swindle and tell fantastic lies (pathological liar).

ETIOLOGY OF PERSONALITY DISORDERS

Psychological factors

Example: early attachments, maladaptive learning.

Constitutional factors

Example: Prenatal factors.

Hereditary factors

Example: Genetic predisposition or chromosomal abnormality such as XYY pattern seen in psychopathy.

Environmental factors

Example: Poverty, low socioeconomic class, broken home.

MANAGEMENT

Personality disorder is often difficult to treat. Drugs are not usually required. Associated mental illness like depression or psychosis can be treated with drugs. Individual or group psychotherapy, therapeutic community and behavioral therapy can be beneficial. Manipulation of the social environment can be tried. There is a tendency to improve naturally with age and maturity.

NURSING CARE OF PATIENT WITH PERSONALITY DISORDERS

Planning and implementing of nursing care for personality disordered clients in one of the greatest challenges in psychiatric mental health nursing. These clients develop an unhealthy negative counter-transparence towards therapist and are difficult to change.

1. Self awareness:
   Develop a high-degree of self awareness.
   Develop emotional control.

   Indicative of negative counter transference
   Anger towards the client defensiveness
   Dominate the client
   } Wanting to control excessive preoccupation with client becoming frustrated, confused and unable to concentrate during interaction.

2. Trust development:
   The nurse need to exercise social care to establish trust
   A straight forward matter of fact approach
   Honesty, respect, and being genuine adds to trust formation
   } Warm approach

   In verbal interaction, nurse should use open-ended questions designed to assist these clients to focus on their behavior and its consequences.

3. Counter-projection:
   When working with a suspicious client, the nurse need to acknowledge that the client's assertions are within the realm of possibility, if not probability, the nurse can then use empathy techniques to encourage the client to talk about real feelings, motives even though they are attributed to others rather than to the self.
4. Time-out:
   Breaking off interaction.
   Postponing the next interaction.

5. Confrontation:

   Confrontation is useful when patient uses manipulation. Pointing out client's problematic behavior helps him to become more self aware. Keys to effective communication are

   Pointing out the behavior as soon as possible after its occurrence.

   Being specific, when describing the behavior.

   Using a non-accusatory, nonjudgmental, matter of fact manner.

   Focusing on the client's actual behavior rather than the client's explanation of it.

6. Limit Setting:

   A client's manipulative, dependent and acting out behavior may necessitate the use of limit setting. Limit setting is more than telling a client to stop a particular behavior. It involves.

   Identify the behavior that client needs to control.

   Offering an appropriate, alternative behavior for client to pursue.

   Anticipate that the client will test nurses to determine if they will back down.

   Remaining steadfast and consistent in the use of limit setting.

   Decrease unacceptable behavior. Establish firm, consistent limits on behavior.

   Improve impulse control. Develop the ability to delay gratification.

   Encourage the verbal expression of frustration.

   Ensuring a safe environment and decreasing the self-mutilating suicidal behavior.

   Help the client to establish supportive relationship with others.

   Help the client to resolve any immediate crisis in his or her life.

   Depending upon the type of personality disorder. Nursing care may vary.

NURSING CARE OF ANTISOCIAL PERSONALITY DISORDER

The long-term goal of nursing care is helping the person to accept responsibility for and consequences of his actions. The short-term goal aims at minimizing manipulation and acting out.

Encourage the patient to talk about his behavior, its limits and consequences.

Discuss how manipulative behavior prevents him from establishing a close relationship.

Help the patient identify more adaptive strategies.

Provide positive feedback for non-manipulative behavior because they cannot be corrected by punishment.

Assist him to understand his positive qualities.

Develop therapeutic rapport with him.

An attitude of acceptance promotes feelings of self-worth.

Trust is the basis of a therapeutic relationship.

Provide group situations for the patient.

Through group interaction, he may learn socially acceptable behavior.

Chapter 14

Mood Disorder (Affective Disorder)

Mood is an internal emotional state of an individual. A mood disorder is characterized by an excessive swing of mood. The mood state of a normal individual fluctuates between mild depressions to mild elation depending on many factors. For example, if she passes an examination, she may be little elated or happy; if she, fails she may be a little depressed or sad. There is also a period to define a mood disorder. It is only when the mood swing is excessive in severity and in duration and when it interferes with a person's day-to-day activities that it becomes a mood disorder.

CLASSIFICATION OF MOOD DISORDERS

Old Term	**New Term**
Manic depressive psychosis	Bipolar disorder
Endogenous depression	Major depression
Neurotic depression	Dysthymic disorder (persistent depressive Disorder (Dysthymia)

MOOD DISORDERS (DEPRESSION AND MANIA)

Primary mood disorder		Secondary mood disorder (depression and mania	
Depressive disorder	Bipolar disorder	Secondary to other psychotic disorder	Secondary to systemic medical disease
Single or recurrent depressive episode	Manic, depressive, mixed	Schizophrenia, dementia, Mixed	CNS disorder endocrine disorders and drug-induced disorder infections

DEPRESSION

Depression is the common cold of psychiatric illness. Very often we come across people saying that they are 'sad', 'depressed', 'down', 'mood out', feeling that they have lost interest in everything and that they are isolated. All these refer to depression. Depression is a mood state. Depression may be a normal mood state if it follows a painful, distressing situation and if it is transient or short-lived. All of us at times feel depressed for a variety of reasons and after some time we come out of that gloom to normal state.

DEPRESSION AS A DISORDER

If depressive mood is very severe in intensity; and if it is going to create problems for the individual and others, if it is going to interfere with the individual's day-to-day activities and if it is prolonged, then this depression is abnormal and a disease. Depression is a very real disease, just like typhoid fever or hypertension. It may come about as reaction to an event, such as the death of a loved one or a change in financial situation, or it may come without any obvious external cause.

EPIDEMIOLOGY

Depression is a widespread mental health problem affecting many people, young and old, rich and poor, men and women. In India, 1-6% of the general population suffers from depression. 5-20% of psychiatric outpatients attending general hospitals suffer from depression.

The common age group is 30-50 years. Depression is more common in old people. In the elderly above 60 years, 13-22 percent suffer from depression. Females suffer more than males. Depression occurs twice as frequently in women as in men. Children and adolescents also suffer from depression, but not as commonly as adults.

MAJOR DEPRESSION

Modern psychiatric classification isolates a syndrome termed major depression. This may be defined as the presence of:

- Depressed mood or
- Loss of interest and pleasure, With 4 or more of the following seven symptoms:
  - Feelings of worthlessness or guilt
  - Impaired concentration
  - Loss of energy and fatigue
  - Thoughts of suicide
  - Loss or increase of appetite and weight
  - Insomnia or excessive sleep and
  - Retardation or agitation.

The above symptoms are required to be present for at least two weeks in the absence of other primary disease. Major depression may be present with or without psychotic features like delusion, hallucination or bizarre behavior.

Persistent Depressive Disorder (PDD)/ Dysthymic Disorder/(Dysthymia)

- Depressed mood for most of the day for at least two years
- Presence of at least two of the following six symptoms:
  - Decreased or increased appetite
  - Decreased or increased sleep
  - Low energy or fatigue
  - Low self-esteem
  - Poor concentration or indecisiveness.

Feelings of hopelessness without any evidence of major depressive disorder for two years and without any other primary disorder.

BIPOLAR DISORDERS

These disorders are characterized by mood swings, from profound depression to extreme euphoria (mania), with intervening periods of normalcy. Bipolar disorders are of three kinds

1. Bipolar disorder
   Mixed (Both manic and depressive episodes intermixed)
2. Bipolar disorder
   Manic (The predominant mood is elevated, expansive or irritable; motor activity is excessive, psychotic features may be evident)
3. Bipolar disorder
   Depressed (Symptoms are characteristic of major depression with a history of at least one manic episode).

MASKED DEPRESSION

In masked depression the patient complains of multiple, vague, bodily symptoms without any other primary disease. Patient may not express a depressed mood state, yet the depression may be underneath or masked and the vague bodily symptoms may be due to an underlying depressive illness.

SEASONAL DEPRESSION

The mood changes that occur during the winter months.

Etiology of Depression

Biological Factors

Genetic factors: Numerous studies have been conducted which support the involvement of heredity in depressive disorders. The incidence of disorder appears to be substantially higher among relatives of individuals with the disorder than among the general population.

Biochemical: Depression is due to the imbalance of biogenic amines in the brain. The amines involved are norepinephrine, serotonin and dopamine. The levels of these amines are reduced in individuals with depressive illness.

Electrolyte imbalance appears to play a role in depressive illness.

An error in metabolism results in the transposition of sodium and potassium. The biochemical theories of depression remain controversial.

Psychological Factors

- Low self-esteem
- Guilt
- Lack of support system
- Lack of clear goals
- Feelings of failure
- Inability to fulfill expectations
- As a response to separation or object loss.

Cognitive narrow negative attitude about self, the environment and the future, bad or inadequate judgments.

Behavioral

- Hopelessness
- Loss of positive reinforcement.

Sociocultural factors

- Social situations that bring feelings of powerlessness and low self-esteem.
- Status of minority group
- Status of women in a male-dominated occupation
- Role loss (Empty nest syndrome)
- Adverse events
- Injustice
- Poverty
- Unemployment.

Alcohol and Depression

There is a strong relationship between alcohol, drug abuse and depression. Alcohol drinking itself may induce depression. People claim that to some extent all alcoholics are depressed. Thus, there exists a cause and effect relationship between alcohol and depression.

Complications of Depression

Some patients with depression recover spontaneously after some time, even without any treatment. But once depression is recognized as an illness it should be actively treated, otherwise there may be the following complications:

- The individual with depressive illness suffers; his work and day-to-day activities suffer and his family suffers as well
- There may be loss in productivity or in the financial status of the individual. Because of his disinterest and incapacitation he may lose his job
- Depression leads on to alcoholism and drug abuse among vulnerable groups
- Depressives are prone to suicide.

Management of Depression

Hospitalization: If the depression is severe and there are suicidal tendencies, it is better to hospitalize the patient for further management.

Drug therapy: With the help of antidepressants, depression can be relieved in a few weeks time. The details regarding drug therapy are given in the chapter on drug treatment (Antidepressant drugs).

Electroconvulsive therapy: It is an effective physical method of treatment in major depression. It is advisable if the depression is severe and with suicidal tendency. ECT is widely used in combination with antidepressant drugs.

Psychotherapy: Psychotherapy means understanding the depressed patients and their problems and guiding them positively. It includes reassurance and supportive measures, and encouraging patients to freely communicate with the therapist. The emotional ventilation has dramatic effect in relieving depression. Family therapy, group therapy and cognitive therapy are also indicated in selected cases of depression. The selection of treatment depends on the individual patients.

Nursing Care in Depression

Promote sleep and food intake—give the prescribed drugs in time and monitor food intake and, if necessary, administer IV fluids.

Assess if there is any suicidal tendency. Take safety measures and keep vigil if patient has suicidal ideas. The patient's safety is a nursing priority.

Diminish feelings of loneliness. Build trust by a one-to-one relationship. Improve interaction with the patient.

The interaction should focus on the present, not the past or far into the future. Reassure the patient that the present depressed mood state is temporary and that he will be protected and helped. Use a kind, firm and warm attitude. The presence of a trusted individual provides emotional security for the patient.

Postpone to your patients decision making and resumption of duties.

Provide non-intellectual activities. For example, cleaning and physical exercise provide safe and effective methods for discharging pent-up tension.

Encourage expression of emotions, denial, hopelessness, helplessness, guilt, etc. Provide the patient the opportunity to cry out and ventilate his anger.

Keep strict records of sleeping patterns. Discourage sleep during the day to promote more restful sleep at night. At night use measures that may promote sleep, such as warm drinks (milk), warm baths, soft music, etc. Limit intake of drinks like coffee, tea and colas. Assist patient in getting to sleep until normal sleep pattern is restored.

Indicate that success is possible and not to be hopeless.

Health Education

Regarding the disease: Educate your depressive patients with the following guidelines:

- Depression is far more common than you might think
- Depression can occur without any obvious external cause, due to biochemical imbalance
- Sometimes the process of getting better takes time and one must wait
- You are not alone; there are many people around you who care about your well-being like your family, your friends and your doctor and his team
- Regarding drugs
- Take your medicines carefully and regularly. Never take less or more than the prescribed dose. Never skip a dose
- Do not expect miracles. It could be at least two weeks before you feel better
- There may be some side effects due to the antidepressants, like dry mouth, constipation, giddiness; do not worry about them
- Some medicines can make you sleep initially and it is good for you to sleep well. Avoid driving or performing any activity which might need a lot of concentration after taking these drugs

- Avoid taking alcohol when you are on medication. They may interact and produce harm
- Do not stop treatment without the doctor's advice
- Advice to family members: Educate the family members in the following ways
- Understand that the patient's problems are due to depression, a disease like any other physical disease and needs active treatment
- Give correct history to the doctor
- Give the medication regularly as prescribed by the doctor
- Give adequate support and encouragement, so that patient may feel more secure and the recovery will be faster
- Watch for any suicidal ideas or gestures and inform your doctor immediately
- Accept him as he is, and give him care and hope.

Nursing care in depression

THERAPEUTIC NEEDS—MEDICATION

Physical Needs

Prevention of suicide
Improve nutrition
Maintenance of personal hygiene
Encourage adequate rest and sleep
Safety of the patient.

Psychosocial Needs

Reduce feelings of dependency and helplessness
Improve self concept
Improve communication
Improve socialization
Reduce a feeling of guilt and apathy.

Recreational Needs

Art, music, dance, and sports.

SPIRITUAL NEEDS

Prayer,
Yoga
Meditation.

DISCHARGE PLAN

Follow-up care.

MANIA

Mania is a mood disorder. It is the name given to the illness when the patient is excessively happy and energetic, Usually mania occurs as a part of bipolar disorder, i.e. mania and depression occurring in cycles (manic depressive psychosis). Very rarely patients get only recurrent attacks of mania alone without any history of depressive episodes.

Mania is now considered either primary or secondary in nature.

Primary mania is an affective or mood disorder.

Secondary mania occurs secondary to a variety of organic disorders. For example, drug intake, infection, neoplasm, epilepsy or metabolic disturbances).

Etiology

Biological factors

Genetic: The incidence of bipolar disorder among relations of affected individuals is higher than in the general population.

Biochemical: Mania is considered to be due to an excess of biogenic amines (norepinephrine or serotonin) in the brain.

Psychological Factors

Faulty dynamics in the family system and disturbed ego development gives way to a strong Id (uncontrollable impulsive behavior). In the psychoanalytic model, mania is viewed as the mirror image of depression—a denial of depression.

The Clinical Features of Mania

A persistently elevated, expansive or irritable mood.

Inflated self-esteem or grandiosity.

Hyperactivity or psychomotor agitation.

Disturbance in sleep—decreased need for sleep.

Pressured speech—more talkative than usual or pressure to keep talking.

Flight of ideas—a subjective experience where thoughts are racing.

Distracted—poor attention span, responds to multiple, unimportant or irrelevant external stimuli.

Excessive involvement in pleasurable activities. For example, excessive spending habit, uninhibited and excessive sexual activity.

Dress is often inappropriate with bright colors that do not match, excessive make-up and jewelry.

Marked impairment in occupational functioning, in social activities or relationships with other.

Different Forms of Mania

If the person is euphoric, elated, dressing colorfully, cracking jokes, talking excessively and overactive, this is labeled as hypomania, a less severe form of mania.

If the person with mania becomes very irritable, excited, violent, and is a nuisance to public, then the condition is labeled as manic excitement.

Management of Mania

Hospitalization: If patient is too excited, is a public nuisance and unable of taking care of himself, then hospitalization is essential.

Drug treatment: To control manic symptoms antipsychotics like haloperidol and chlorpromazine can be used. Injection haloperidol 5–10 mg IM 2 hours by till the patient is sedated or, maximum of 50 mg (rapid neuroleptization) and change to tablet haloperidol 1.5 to 10 mg three times a day.

OR

Injection chlorpromazine 50–100 mg IM to start with, followed by tablet chlorpromazine 100–200 mg three times a day and to be reduced gradually. Both haloperidol and chlorpromazine tablets can be combined. For patients, who suffer from frequent relapses lithium is best indicated. Lithium is an antimanic and a preventive drug. It is a mood stabilizer. Carbamazepine and sodium valproate can also be given in addition to antipsychotics. ECT may be considered in manic excitement.

Nursing Care of Manic Patient

The person suffering from manic disorder is an overactive individual with an excessive amount of energy. The patient is easily stimulated mentally and physically. The patient may react to this stimulation by constantly being excited, domineering, irritable or vulgar. His attention is easily distracted. Feelings of aggression and hostility are directed outward, to the environment. The overactive patient might be extremely likeable, talkative and euphoric.

Therapeutic Needs—Medication

Physical Needs

- Reduce physical activities and provides adequate sleep
- Improve diet and fluid intake
- Protect the patient from injury to self and others
- Reduce verbal activity
- Pursue the patient to attend to personal hygiene.

Psychosocial Needs

- Improve judgment
- Improve attention and concentration
- Improve communication
- Appropriate socialization
- Realistic self-concept.

Diet: Special attention must be given to the patient's diet because he is usually too busy to eat and hence may lose weight and dehydration may occur. Meals and fluids are to be given under supervision. Extra nourishment may be required to compensate for extra activity.

Medications: Drugs are of great help in dealing with problems of restlessness, sleeplessness and fatigue associated with overactivity.

Others

Supervision is necessary for adequate nutrition and rest.

Bursts of excitement and destructive actively may result in injuries. Therefore, they should be observed and attended.

Supervision and directions to maintain personal hygiene like bathing, oral hygiene are essential.

Care to be taken that the patient is dressed appropriately.

Emotional needs: Frequent mood changes and excitement may be there. Approach the patient in a calm, unhurried and consistent manner. Always speak quietly, tactfully and patiently. Avoid arguments, discussions or situations that are stimulating and irritating.

Suggestions and persuasion are more effective.

One nurse should establish rapport with one overactive patient and improve his confidence in her.

Short, simple direct answers should be quietly given when the patient asks questions.

Maintain a low level of stimuli in the patient's environment.

Observe the patient's behavior frequently. Remove all dangerous objects from patient's environment, so that in his or her hyperactive, agitated state they cannot be used to harm self or others.

Maintaining a therapeutic environment: The ward must be quiet and pleasant. Factors that irritate the patient like excessive noise, bright colors, etc. are to be avoided. Separate rooms may be ideal with simple furnishing. Fluctuation of mood states must be watched. Active games, ward occupation and creative work will channelize his energy. Drug therapy is essential for sedation.

Chapter

15

Schizophrenia

Schizophrenia is a major mental disorder. It is the most common of the psychotic disorders. It has been estimated that 50 percent of all mental hospital beds are occupied by patients diagnosed as schizophrenic.

The word schizophrenic is derived from a Greek word schizo (split) and phrenic (mind).

The term schizophrenia was first coined by a Swiss psychiatrist Eugen Bleuler. Schizoprenia indicates a group of disturbances which sometimes occur in different combinations and intensities. Hence, it is heterogeneous in nature. Schizophrenia has generally been considered to be of ancient origin.

DEFINITION

Schizophrenia is defined as a functional psychosis characterized by disturbances in thinking, emotion, volition and perception. Finally, it leads on to personality deterioration. The illness occurs in a state of clear consciousness. Unlike many psychological disorders, schizophrenia often incapacitates a person. People suffering from schizophrenia display sudden changes in mood, thought, perception and overall behavior. These changes are often accompanied by distortions of reality.

EPIDEMIOLOGY

Schizophrenia is a common disease prevalent in all cultures and in all parts of the world. Three to four per 1000 in any community suffer from schizophrenia. About one percent of the general population stand the risk of this disease in their lifetime. About two-thirds of the cases are in the 15 to 30 years age group. The disease is more common in the lower social classes.

ETIOLOGY

How or why schizophrenia develops remains a puzzle despite extensive research. Current views indicates that it is most likely to be a breakdown in the balance between three interacting sets of factors, namely, biological, psychological and social.

GENETIC FACTORS

The case for a genetic basis of schizophrenic disorders has been supported by a variety of studies, including adoptional studies and twin studies. Such studies lend support to the hypothesis that genetic factors play an important role in the causation of schizophrenia, which probably varies from person to person.

Incidence of schizophrenia in specific populations:

Population	Incidence (%)
General population	1.0
Sibling of schizophrenic patient	8.0
Child with one schizophrenic parent	12.0
Dizygotic twin of a schizophrenic patient	12.0
Child of two schizophrenic parents	40.0
Monozygotic twin of a schizophrenic patient	47.0

BIOCHEMICAL FACTORS

The idea of the physical basis of schizophrenia is not new. A number of biochemical theories have been put forth as the probable cause for schizophrenia, but nothing has proved to be confirmative, although, there are some important theories.

Dopamine Hypothesis

It is based on the idea that the mechanism of action of antipsychotic drugs can shed light on the psychotic disorders they treat. Antipsychotic drugs block postsynaptic dopamine receptor sites in the brain. This led to the speculation that schizophrenia might involve excessive levels of dopamine as a neurotransmitter.

Transmethylation Hypothesis

Schizophrenia may result from abnormal transmethylation of catecholamines.

Indolamine Hypothesis

A defect in the metabolism of indolamine, most probably serotonin, is being investigated as a possible cause of schizophrenia.

According to the biological view as the cause of schizophrenia, the environment triggers this behavior in people who are predisposed to it. Thus, for those who opt for the combined view of nature and nurture, genetic abnormalities lead to situation in which environmental stressors trigger the behavioral pattern of schizophrenia.

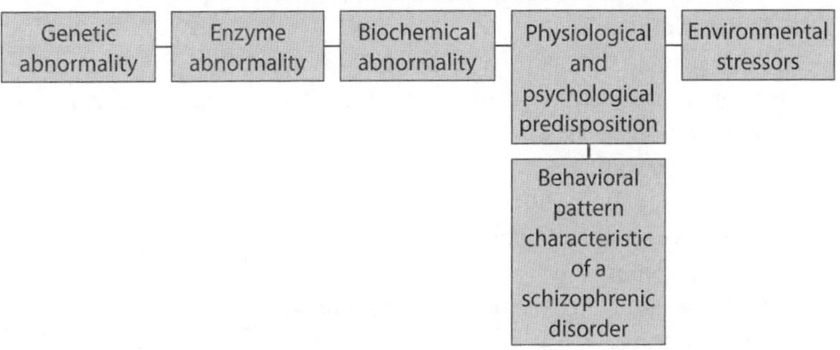

PSYCHOLOGICAL FACTORS

Persons who are withdrawn and have very few social contacts (introverted personalities or schizoid personalities) are more prone to develop schizophrenic illness.

Ego boundary disturbance is also considered to be a cause of schizophrenia. Behaviorists assert that negative reinforcement and extinction schedules cause schizophrenia. Most psychoanalysts and behavioral theories suggest that a person's relationship to the environment can bring about schizophrenia. Freud believed that schizophrenic patients regress to a phase of primary narcissism and ego disintegration.

SOCIAL OR ENVIRONMENTAL FACTORS

Children and adults develop schizophrenia because their home environment is not conducive to normal emotional growth. People who have developed schizophrenia tend to come from families where there is considerable conflict. Generally, communication between parents and children in such families is inadequate. There is communication deviance.

Some studies have shown that schizophrenia is more prevalent in areas of high social mobility and disorganization, especially, in members of very low social class.

CLINICAL FEATURES

There are four groups of symptoms

- Positive
- Negative
- Cognitive
- Affective (Mood)
- Other

1. Positive symptoms
   For example, delusions, hallucinations, bizarre behavior, suspicious, over activity, aggression, agitation and hostility.
2. Negative symptoms
   Apathy, avolition (Lack of will power), social withdrawal, diminished emotional responsiveness, blunted affect, stereotyped thinking, lack of spontaneity.
3. Cognitive symptoms
   Memory problems, difficulty in thinking, difficulty in planning, inadequate decision making and improper judgment.
4. Affective symptoms
   Depression, guilt, anxiety and perplex emotions.
5. Other symptoms:
   - Thought disturbance is the predominant disturbance in schizophrenia.
   - Persons suffering from schizophrenia will have poor personal hygiene; sleep disturbance, behavior problem like bizarre mannerisms, negativism, stupor or at times excitement.
   - Lack of insight, i.e. not aware that he or she is suffering from an illness. It is one of the cardinal symptoms of schizophrenia.

- First rank symptoms
  - Audible thoughts
  - Voices arguing or discussing or both
  - Voices commenting
  - Somatic passivity experiences
  - Thought withdrawal and other experiences of influenced thought
  - Thought broadcasting
  - Delusional perceptions
  - All other experiences involving volition made affects, and made impulses.
- Second rank symptoms
  - Other disorders of perception
  - Sudden delusional ideas
  - Perplexity
  - Depressive and euphoric mood changes
  - Feelings of emotional impoverishment
  - And several others as well.

TYPES OF SCHIZOPHRENIA

- Paranoid schizophrenia—**prominent symptoms are delusions and hallucinations.**

- Hebephrenic schizophrenia (Disorganized type)—**essential features are marked incoherence and flat, incongruous or silly affect.**
- Catatonic schizophrenia—**the clinical feature is dominated by psychomotor disturbance. This includes rigidity, stupor, negativism or excitement.**
- Residual schizophrenia—**currently no prominent symptoms; but history of one episode with prominent symptoms should be there.**
- Undifferentiated schizophrenia—**the psychotic symptoms here cannot be classified in any category.**
- Simple schizophrenia—**progressive symptoms with odd behavior, wandering tendency and aimless activity very poor prognosis.**

If schizophrenia exists continuously for more than 2 years, we call that as chronic schizophrenia.

MANAGEMENT OF SCHIZOPHRENIA

Management includes:

1. Drug treatment (Psychopharmacology)
2. Psychological methods of treatment like counseling, psychotherapy, family therapy, group therapy and behavior modification.
3. Rehabilitation which aims at trying to make the individual to live a near normal life inspite of the disability.

DRUG TREATMENT FOR SCHIZOPHRENIA

The drugs used to reduce the symptoms of schizophrenia are known as antipsychotics. Some of the common drugs used are

Drugs	Class
Haloperidol Trifluperazine Chlorpromazine	Conventional antipsychotics (First generation antipsychotics)
Clozapine Risperidone Olanzapine Quetiapine	Atypical antipsychotics (Second generation antipsychotics)

Amisulpride
Aripiprazole
Risperidone
Zotepine.

- Second generation and antipsychotics (Atypical) are preferred as the first line of management

- In the acute phase—injection haloperidol 10–30 mg in divided doses may be beneficial
- For long-term maintenance long-acting injection like injection haloperidol long-acting 25 mg once in 2 to 4 week can be used.

Comprehensive care of the chronic schizophrenia includes drug treatment and other psychological methods of treatment with long-term rehabilitation.

Psychological Methods of Treatment

Psychosocial therapies include: Individual, group and family psychotherapy. CBT is necessary. Rehabilitation is vital along with drug treatment for better out come.

NURSING CARE OF SCHIZOPHRENIA

First, the nurse should understand the following general principle of management of schizophrenic patients.

Schizophrenia is a chronic illness, hence, the maintenance of long-term treatment is essential. Total cure may not be possible in most of the cases.

What one should aim at is good improvement, with regular, appropriate treatment.

Furthermore, in times of stress, the patient may get a relapse of symptoms inspire of regular treatment.

A schizophrenic patient requires a substantial increase in his own self-esteem. Needs to be assisted to live with the real world.

Needs to live in a place where he gets a change to use his own initiative and judgment.

Needs to have human contacts.

Needs to find a nurse who will be a stable and consistent model. He needs assurance as to his own personal identity. Needs patience, and forbearance.

Accept him as he is. That means the nurse should realize the limitations and weaknesses of the patient.

The nurse can minimize her own frustrations by learning not to expect the impossible from him. The patient's condition can be made to improve, but slowly. Hence, it is the duty of the nurse to refrain from rejecting him and accepting him wholeheartedly as he is.

Assign small responsibilities to the patient.

Engage and support the patient.

Supervise him in all his needs.

Appreciate him even if he does a small task.

Do not—Ignore
Criticize
Exert social behavior
Refrain from over-involvement.

Secondly, a careful assessment should be made to provide diagnosis and to confirm or to help to formulate a treatment plan.

The nursing management needs may vary from defining reality, handling patient control, strengthening the patient's self-image and strengthening the interpersonal relationship.

By giving emotional support, the patient can incorporate positive feelings and feel good about himself. Thus, he will have a strong chance to be able to return to the community to lead a normal life again.

The nurse should use the skills and techniques appropriate to the specific therapy.

Nursing Care of the Acutely Ill Schizophrenics

Schizophrenic patients may become acutely ill, mostly during the initial stage of the illness or they may get acute exacerbations during their long-term course of the illness. Acute excitements are more common in catatonic and paranoid types. The main nursing concern is controlling his impulsive behavior, when he hears voices and responds to them. He will be also verbally abusive to the staff. It may be difficult to communicate with someone who is psychotic, but it is important to obtain valuable data on how severe the thought disorder is. These data can be obtained by the nurse who can establish some degree of trust with the patient.

During the acute phase, the most important thing is to meet the physical need of the patient.

Proper nutritional care is essential since the patient may refuse food because of suspicion, indifference (negligence) or too busy or over-active that he forgets to take food.

So, it is important to supervise the patient's nutrition and if necessary, intravenous fluids will be given to avoid dehydration. In the acute phase, schizophrenic patients require drugs mainly by parenteral form. For example, injection chlorpromazine 100 mg intramuscular, injection haloperidol 10 to 20 mg intramuscular or intravenous. The injections are to be continued periodically till the patient is able to take oral drugs. During acute state, it is important to look for any injuries sustained during excitement and these should be attended to. The acutely excited patients should always be approached with the assistance of other nursing staff or attenders.

Nursing Care of the Chronic Schizophrenics

Schizophrenia is a disease which is chronic in nature and the chronic patients are usually withdrawn and have a lot of negative symptoms. So, very important in the nursing care of chronic schizophrenics is to engage the patient in some useful activity. "An idle mind is the devil's workshop", therefore, the patient who lives in a fantasy will have a poor prognosis. Patients will lose their original potentials, yet, they will have some minimum capabilities.

To make him lead a beneficial life with the existing potential, he should be encouraged to do some positive, physical work. This is otherwise known as rehabilitation. It is the role of the nurse to encourage and motivate the patient to have some occupation or to work in some industrial therapeutic unit. The nurse should also constantly supervise the patient's performance and appreciate him at the appropriate time.

Following are physical, emotional and therapeutical needs of the chronic patients.

Physical Needs

- Appropriate nutrition-regular diet and supervision of his diet
- Taking care of personal hygiene-regular bath and cleanliness.

Elimination has to be carefully watched-attend to care of the skin because a chronic schizophrenic living in a crowded, closed place are prone to develop skin problems like scabies, eczema, etc.

Emotional Needs

- The withdrawn patient's main problem is lack of communication and poor interpersonal relationship because of less social contact.
- It is the responsibility of the nurse to improve his communication and also his social contacts by encouraging the relatives/friends to visit him often.
- It is also the responsibility of the nurse to give importance to the personal identity of the patient.

Therapeutic Needs

He should be accepted as a human being and should be given responsible work in the ward set-up. Patiently and positively hear the suggestions from the patient himself in implementing the routine ward work. This type of therapeutic environment will minimize the damage and will improve the quality of the person. This will again prevent **institutional neurosis**—a condition which may occur in a long-term mentally ill patient in a mental hospital set-up.

The chronic patient needs stimulation, occupational, and recreational therapies.

In the nursing care of a chronic schizophrenic, emphasis should be placed on the five "R"s

- Reassurance
- Readjustment
- Reeducation
- Rehabilitation
- Recreation.

Psychosocial Needs

- Decreased disturbed thoughts
- Reduce delusions
- Decrease hallucination
- Improve communication
- Improve socialization
- Enhance self concept
- Improve attention and judgment
- Improve family support.

Physical Needs

- Prevent from injury
- Personal hygiene needs
- Improve sleep
- Nutritional needs.

Recreational Needs

Art, music, dance, and sports.

Spiritual Needs

- Prayer
- Yoga
- Meditation.

Discharge Plan

Follow-up in next 15 to 20 days.

Chapter

16

The Abuse of Alcohol and Drugs

From time immemorial, human beings have looked for substances to make life more pleasurable and to avoid or decrease pain, discomfort, and frustration. Despite definite improvements in health care in most countries, problems related to drug and alcohol abuse are increasing almost everywhere.

Drug use is abnormal, if it causes disturbances, such as:

- When it interferes with normal activities
- Causes physical damage
- Leads to social disapproval.

Drug abuse has been showing a rising trend all over the world including India as a result of newer and greater stresses related to rapid changes in lifestyles. Various terminologies are used in this area like drug abuse, drug addiction and drug dependence—all denoting a basic problem with some differences.

Drug abuse: Drug abuse is defined as persistent or sporadic drug use inconsistent with, or unrelated to, acceptable medical practice.

Drug addiction: A disease process characterized by the continued use of a specific psychoactive substance despite physical, psychological or social harm. Addiction usually indicates a more serious problem than abuse.

Drug dependence: A maladaptive pattern of substance use leading to significant impairment or distress as manifested by the following:

1. Tolerance
   A need for markedly increased amounts of the substance in order to achieve intoxication or desired effect.
2. Characteristic withdrawal symptoms
   If the abused drug is stopped or reduced in quantity, the person develops physical and/or psychological disturbances.
3. Frequent preoccupation with seeking or taking the substance.
4. Often takes the substance in larger amounts or over a longer period than was intended.

5. Often takes the substance to relieve or avoid withdrawal symptoms.
6. There are unsuccessful efforts to cut down or control substance use.
7. Much time is spent in search of, or to obtain, the drug.
8. Important social, occupational or recreational activities are given up or reduced because of substance use.
9. Intoxicated by substance when expected to attend to his duties (e.g. does not go to work because of hangover; goes to work high; drives when drunk).
10. Continuation of substance use despite a significant occupational, social or legal problem or a physical disorder.

TYPES OF ABUSED SUBSTANCES

Types of Substances

Examples
Effects
Depressants
Alcohol, barbiturates, sedatives, sleeping tablets
Drowsiness, pleasant relaxation, disinhibition
Opiates
Morphine, methadone, Heroin
Relief from pain, pleasant, detached feeling, euphoria
Stimulants
Cocaine,
Amphetamines
Exhilaration, reduced fatigue and hunger
Hallucinogens
LSD, Mescaline
Other worldliness, perceptual distortions
Cannabis
Marijuana, ganja,
Bhang
Relaxation, and
hallucinogenic effects
Nicotine
Tobacco
Sedation and stimulation
Volatile inhalants
Glues, paint thinners
Drowsiness, relaxation,
perceptual disturbances.

ALCOHOL ABUSE

Even though, alcohol is a depressant, it will be considered separately due to the complex effects and widespread nature of its use. Alcoholism is defined as a chronic disease manifested by repeated drinking that produces injury to the drinker's health or to his social or economic functioning.

Low-to-moderate consumption produces a feeling of well-being and reduced inhibitions. At higher concentrations, motor and intellectual functions are impaired, mood becomes very labile and behavior characteristic of depression, euphoria and aggression are exhibited. The medical use of alcohol is:

1. As an ingredient in medicines in some pharmacological preparations like cough syrup, tonics, etc.
2. As an antidote for methanol consumption.

Alcoholic beverages are widely used in many societies because of which their abuse potential is often underestimated. Commonly used alcohol preparations are beer, wine, brandy, whisky, rum, gin, arrack and toddy.

Alcoholism is the most common psychiatric disorder. Epidemiological surveys carried out in India reveal that 20 to 40 percent of subjects aged above 15 are current users of alcohol and nearly, 10 percent of them are regular or excessive users. Nearly 15 to 30 percent of patients seeking admission in psychiatric facilities are for alcohol-related problems. Among the acute medical admissions in a general hospital, 10 to 20 percent are due to alcohol-related problems.

The Causes of Alcohol Abuse

Availability: Alcohol is easily available and drinking is accepted as a 'norm' in functions and social gathering.

Genetic factors: Some excessive drinkers have a family history of excessive drinking. There is a genetic relation between alcoholism, depression and antisocial personality disorder.

Biochemical factors: Several biochemical factors have been suggested including abnormalities in alcohol dehydrogenase or in the neurotransmitter mechanism.

Learned behavior: It has been suggested that learning process may contribute in a more specific way to the development of alcohol dependence through the repeated experience of withdrawal symptoms.

Alcohol may act as a reinforcer for further drinking. Children especially boys, tend to follow their parents' drinking pattern. Some people drink to get away from pain.

Personality factors: Alcoholism is more common in anxiety, prone or cyclothymic personalities. Drinking alcohol is also more common among antisocial personalities.

Poor coping strategies: The person unable to face stress often resort to alcoholism. The defense mechanisms involved in alcoholism include denial, rationalization and projection.

Psychiatric disorders: Some patients with depressive disorders take alcohol in the mistaken hope that it will alleviate low mood. Persons suffering from anxiety disorders and phobic disorders are prone to take alcohol as an escape.

Social causes: Isolation, unemployment, loss, injustice and other social causes may lead to alcoholism.

High risk groups: Persons suffering from chronic physical illness, business executives, traveling salespersons, industrial workers, urban slum dwellers, students in hostels, military personnel, etc. are more prone to develop alcohol abuse.

THE PROCESS OF DEVELOPMENT OF ALCOHOLISM

Experimental: To begin with, persons start drinking alcohol due to peer pressure and curiosity.

Recreational: Gradually, whenever, they meet in functions like marriages, hostel day or college day, parties, conferences, they drink occasionally.

Relaxational: Further, whenever, they want relaxation on holidays and weekends, they start enjoying their drink and continue to do so. Hence, the frequency gradually increases.

Compulsive: Some people who started drinking occasionally, start drinking almost daily or drinking heavily for a period of time for pleasure or to avoid the discomfort of withdrawal symptoms.

The disease goes through distinct stages:

Early Stage

Increased tolerance—needing more and more of alcohol to experience the same pleasure as experienced earlier.

Blackouts—inability to recollect incidents which happened under the influence of alcohol.

Preoccupation—always thinking about how, when and where to drink.

Middle Stage

Loss of control over amount, time and occasion of drinking. Keeping away from alcohol for some time, but going back, obsessive drinking after each such abstinent period.

Chronic Stage

Getting drunk even on small amounts of alcohol.
Willing to lie, beg, borrow or steal to maintain supply of alcohol.
Living to drink—alcohol takes priority over family or job.

PHYSICAL COMPLICATIONS OF ALCOHOL ABUSE

Gastrointestinal

- Dyspepsia
- Vomiting
- Acute or chronic gastritis
- Peptic ulcer
- Cancer.

Liver

- Fatty degeneration of the liver
- Alcoholic hepatitis
- Cirrhosis.

Pancreas

- Acute and chronic pancreatitis.

Cardiovascular

- Alcoholic cardiomyopathy
- High risk for myocardial infarction.

Blood

- Folic acid deficiency anemia
- Decreased WBC production.

Muscle

- Peripheral muscle weakness
- Wasting of muscles.

Skin

- Spider angiomas
- Acne.

Nutrition

- Protein malnutrition
- Vitamin deficiency disorders like pellagra and beriberi.

Joints

- Gout due to increase in uric acid level.

Reproductive System

- Sexual dysfunction in males
- Failure of ovulation in females.

Pregnancy

- Fetal alcohol syndrome—fetal abnormalities like mental retardation and growth deficiency.

Nervous System

- Alcoholic peripheral neuropathy
- Wernicke's-Korsakoff syndrome
- Rum fits during withdrawal.

PSYCHIATRIC COMPLICATIONS OF ALCOHOL ABUSE

Pathological intoxication: Maladaptive behavioral effects, such as fighting, impaired judgment, physiological signs such as slurred speech, incoordination, and unsteady gait. Psychological changes such as mood changes, irritability, and impaired attention.

Withdrawal phenomenon: The general withdrawal symptoms are—tremor, nausea and vomiting, malaise, tachycardia, elevated blood pressure, irritability, anorexia, insomnia, fits.

Delirium tremens (DT): It is a complicated withdrawal state. An acute organic mental disorder should be treated as a psychiatric emergency. DT is a short-lived, but occasionally life-threatening, toxic, confusional state with accompanying somatic disturbance. Prodromal symptoms are insomnia, tremulousness and fear, and occasionally convulsions. The classical features are:

a. Clouding of consciousness and confusion.
b. Vivid visual hallucinations and illusions.
c. Marked tremor and fever.
d. Delusion, agitation, increased ANS activities.

Alcoholic hallucinosis: Vivid hallucinations developing shortly after cessation or reduction of alcohol.

Alcoholic psychosis: Person drinking alcohol for a long time and in large quantities is prone to develop a psychotic disorder which resembles a paranoid schizophrenia with clinical features like behavioral problem, thought disturbance, delusions and impairment of primary mental functions.

Morbid jealousy (Othello syndrome): A paranoid disorder with predominant delusion of infidelity of spouse (Suspecting wife's character).

Alcoholism and depression: Alcoholics are more prone to develop depression. To get relief from depression some people will further aggravate the depression. Attempted suicides are more common in alcoholics.

Alcoholism and criminality: Alcohol reduces inhibition and increases hostile behavior. Hence, alcoholics are more prone to violence and antisocial behavior.

Alcoholism and sex: Alcohol increases the sexual desire away but takes away the performance. Alcoholic males suffer from sexual dysfunction.

Alcohol amnestic disorder: Impairment in short- and long-term memory with disorientation and confabulation.

Alcoholic dementia: A chronic organic mental disorder due to long-term alcohol drinking. Irreversible impairment in memory, orientation, impulse control, ability to solve problems, etc. may be there.

SOCIAL COMPLICATIONS OF ALCOHOLISM

Work Problems: Decreased work performance, hence decreased productivity due to chronic absences. As a result, the economy of the nation suffers.

Family Problems: Alcoholism is a disease which not only affects the individuals, but his whole family. Loss of job, loss of income will make the family condition miserable. There will be a role model reversal, i.e. the bread-winner becomes an alcoholic and the wife takes the role of earning. Marital disharmony is a common complication.

Drunken Driving: Will lead to accidents.

MANAGEMENT OF ALCOHOLISM

- Assessment of the patient
  - His drinking pattern
  - Work spot
  - Family
  - Environment.
- Physical methods
  - Detoxification.
  - Disulfiram therapy.
- Psychological methods
  - Counseling
  - Individual and group psychotherapy
  - Military and family therapy
  - Behavioral modification (aversion therapy)
  - Relapse prevention therapy.
- Rehabilitation
- Alcoholic anonymous.

Detoxification: Detoxification is the process by which an alcohol dependent person recovers from the intoxicating effects of alcohol in a supervised way. It includes:

Administration of minor tranquilisers (antianxiety drugs like chlordiazepoxide or diazepam) to control anxiety, insomnia, agitation and tremors.

Assess fluid and electrolyte balance for dehydration—IV fluids are essential.

Re-establish proper nutrition by giving a diet high in protein (when there is no liver damage), carbohydrate, vitamins C and B-complex (especially vitamin B1, B6 and B12) preparation parenterally. Provide calm, safe environment, control nausea and vomiting, and administer anticonvulsants if there is withdrawal seizure (rumfit).

Disulfiram (Antabuse) therapy: This drug produces intense headaches, severe flushing, extreme nausea, vomiting, palpitations, hypotension, dyspnea and blurred vision, when alcohol is consumed by the person.

Aversion therapy: Patient is subjected to pain-inducing stimuli at the time of drinking to establish alcohol-rejection behavior.

Alcoholics Anonymous (AA): A self group of ex-addicts who confront, instruct and support fellow-drinkers in their efforts to stay sober one day at a time, through fellowship and acceptance.

NURSING CARE OF ALCOHOL DEPENDENTS

The nurse taking care of an alcoholic in a de-addiction ward should understand some basic concepts about the problem:

1. Alcoholism is a chronic disorder.
2. It is a relapsing disorder.
3. It is a disease, affecting physical, mental and social well-being.
4. Not only does the individual suffer, but his family, work and community also suffer.
5. Accepting drinking as a problem by the patient is an important first step, because most of the alcoholics deny that they are addicts (denial).
6. They are prone to pathological lying and manipulative behavior.
7. The involvements of other significant persons, especially, the family members enhance the recovery process.

The Important Five Goals in the Management of Alcoholism Include

1. Improving social relationships and supports.
2. Developing confidence and ability to change.
3. Identifying reasons to change.
4. Developing alternative activities.
5. Learning to prevent relapse.

Care in the Acute Stage (Immediately after admission during detoxification)

- Patient to be kept in a quiet environment
- Excessive stimuli increase the patient's agitation. Well-lighted rooms help reduce fears and illusions
- Safety precautions-careful observation of the patient's behavior
- Observe for any sign of developing Delirium tremens (DT)
- Be sure that the side-rails are up when the patient is in bed
- Physical restraint may be necessary if patient is highly disturbed or hyperactive
- Keep potentially harmful objects away from the room since the chance of deliberate self harm is there
- Keep the bed clean, dry and warm since some patients may be incontinent
- Monitor vital signs every 15 minutes initially
- Frequently orient the patient to reality and surroundings.

Medication

- Follow medication as advised by the doctor
- Antianxiety drugs like chlordiazepoxide (Librium) and diazepam, if necessary, parenterally given
- Plenty of vitamins, especially injection B1, B6 and B12 and tablet B complex and vitamin C
- Antacids to relieve gastritis
- Correct fluid and electrolyte imbalance by IV fluids.

Nutrition

- Take care of the nutrition of the patient
- Document intake, output and calorie content
- Weigh daily
- Ensure that the patient receives small frequent feedings rather than large meals
- Ask family members to bring food that the patient enjoys.

Delirium tremens (DT): It is an acute organic mental disturbance during the withdrawal period of alcoholism. Watch for symptoms like confusion, disorientation, tremor, illusion, hallucination, agitation and apprehension and increased sweating, heart beat and pulse rate. Some patients may throw fit (Rum fit). DT should be treated as emergency since it may sometimes be fatal. IV fluid and IV diazepam, keeping the patient in quiet room, supplement with B complex vitamins and reassurance are essential.

Nursing Care during Later Stage of Hospitalization (After Detoxification is Over)

- To understand the alcoholic, it is important to look beyond the symptoms and learn about the person. These persons are in need of physical as well as social rehabilitation
- Attention to their rest, diet, personal hygiene and appearance is important
- During the recovery and rehabilitation period, the acceptance of the patient by the nurse is essential. The nurse's acceptance may encourage the patient to socialize and participate in planned ward activities
- The alcoholic patients have inferior feelings and low self-esteem, If the nurse accepts him as an individual and cordially talks to him, these feelings will be reduced
- The nurse should be empathetic with the person, but should not be over-sympathetic and be sure that they do not become dependent on her

- The nurse has an important role in the care and rehabilitation of alcoholic patients and their families. The wives should always be included in the psychological therapy
- It is important for the nurse to anticipate improvement instead of complete cure
- Expression of kindness and being nonjudgmental, accepting him, being consistent and understanding in approach, all induces a favorable relationship, which will help the recovery process.

Nurses Role in the Prevention of Alcohol Abuse

Primary prevention: Aim to avoid the appearance of new cases of alcohol abuse by reducing the consumption of alcohol through health promotion, especially health education.

Secondary prevention: Attempt to detect cases early, and to treat them before serious complications cause disability.

Tertiary prevention: Aim to avoid further disabilities and to reintegrate individuals into society who have been harmed by severe alcohol-related problems.

The nurse will be involved in all of these levels.
Detoxification: This means to withdraw the intake of alcohol controlling the withdrawal symptoms.

Patient might experience delirium tremens when alcohol is withdrawn.
Special attention to be provided.
Provide adequate nutrition and prevent dehydration.

Physical care for the safety of the patient.

1. Psychotherapy.
2. Group support therapy.
3. Relaxation exercises.
4. Behavior modification.
5. Aversion therapy disulfiram.
6. Antabuse therapy.
7. Rehabilitation.
8. Alcoholic anonymous.
9. Religious support groups.
10. Health education to the patient and family members.

DRUG ABUSE

Drug abuse was considered a problem in the West, but now, it is a serious public health and socioeconomic problem in India as well. Drug abuse is increasing among Indian youth. Drug addiction is spreading to all sections of the society, especially, high in major cities. It is estimated that 10–25 percent of college students take drugs for euphoria and 1–2 percent abuse drugs. The problem of drug addiction is more common in urban slum dwellers, especially unemployed youth. In India 19–23 per 1000 abuse drugs in the general population.

Drug addiction is neither delinquency nor deviancy, but is a disease worse than cancer. It is a disease because it affects physical health, mental health, prestige, finance, social status and occupation of the individual.

Why People Take Drugs?

- The search for euphoria (a sense of wellbeing)
- Relief of psychological pain of diverse origins
- Wanting to feel better than they do
- To avoid withdrawal symptoms.

The Factors Involved in Drug Abuse

1. The drug is seen as a reinforcer.
2. Tolerance.
3. Physical dependence.
4. The abuser
   - The personality, degree of stability and attitude of the individual.
5. The environment
   - Isolation
   - Stress
   - Peer group influence.
6. The motivating factors
   - Initiation by company
   - Curiosity
   - Pleasure
   - Acceptance by the group.

Identification of an Addict

It is possible to identify the early signs and symptoms of addiction. They are:

- Lack of interest in studies and poor academic performance
- Loss of interest in hobbies games and sports
- Withdrawal from the family
- Social isolation, prefering to be aloof
- Blank expression and irresponsible and aggressive behavior
- Irregular eating and sleeping habits
- Long hours in the bathroom

- Persistent lying and stealing
- Lack of energy and motivation
- Low productivity
- Impaired judgment.

Common Drugs Abused in Our Country

1. Alcohol (dealt in detail already).
2. Cannabis (Ganja).
3. Opium products.
   - Brown sugar (heroin).
   - Synthetic preparations.
4. Hypnotic and minor tranquilizers (diazepam, nitrazepam, etc).

Cannabis: It is the generic name given to the drug containing plant products of Indian hemp. This plant material contains psychoactive chemicals, the most important of which is tetrahydrocannabinol (THC). The dried leaves or flowering tops are often referred to as ganja or marijuana.

The resin of the plant is referred to as hashish.

Bhang is a drink made from cannabis produces psychological dependence.

The psychiatric Complications of Cannabis Abuse

1. Intoxication: Tachycardia, euphoria, perceptual intensification, apathy, relaxation, drowsiness, anxiety, suspiciousness, increased appetite, dry mouth, conjunctival infection. On overdose, it produces confusion, disorientation, panic and hallucination.
2. Flashback: The re-experience of perceptual symptoms that occurred during acute intoxification.
3. Cannabis induced psychosis: A psychosis resembling paranoiac schizophrenia. Clinical features include persecutory ideas or delusions, auditory hallucinations, anxiety, apprehension, suspicion, severe depersonalization, derealization and at times acute depression.
4. Cannabis induced chronic conditions:
   - Personality deterioration
   - Cognitive functional disturbance
   - Sexual dysfunction
   - Social withdrawal
   - Amotivational syndrome (apathy-inactivity, self neglect and nonproductivity).

The common physical complaint associated with Cannabis abuse is bronchitis.

Opioids (Narcotics)

Commonly abused narcotics in our country are brown sugar (heroin) and synthetic preparations like pethidine, Fortwin (pentazocine) and tidigesic (buprenorphine). The abuse of unrefined heroin has spread rapidly in recent years among city-based slum youths. Besides sale of these illegal drugs, other forms of crime and violence increase as this drug abuse spreads.

India is surrounded by countries with a high cultivation of poppy plants and India has emerged as a major transit point for drug trafficking in the region.

Opium is the resin obtained from the poppy plant and contains psychoactive substances like morphine, heroin and codeine (commonly used drug for relieving pain and cough).

In the recent past in our country, the prevalence of injecting drug users were increasing day by day, especially in the urban slum dwelling unemployed youth. At present, majority of the heroin users are administering it by needles. The drugs that are used by needle are—heroin, buprenorphine and pentazocine. Though most opiate users had begun chasing (inhaling the smoke) of heroin they gradually shifted to needle use (Fixing). These injecting drug users have become a high risk group for HIV infection and now play a major role in the transmission of HIV.

The Psychiatric Complications of Narcotics

Intoxication: Euphoria, apathy, psychomotor retardation, drowsiness, slurred speech, constricted pupils, nausea, impaired judgment, relief of pain are the usual effects.

The effects of overdose are, slow and shallow breathing, clammy skin, convulsions, coma and possibly death.

Withdrawal Symptoms

Narcotic withdrawal rarely produces a life-threatening situation.

It includes watery eyes, running nose, yawning, loss of appetite, irritability, tremors, panic, chills (goose flesh), sweating, cramps. nausea, dilated pupils; diarrhea, insomnia and elevated temperature, pulse, respiration and blood pressure.

Withdrawal symptoms of narcotics begin within 12 hours of the last dose. It peaks in 24-36 hours, subsides in 72 hours and disappears in 5-6 days.

Nursing Care of Drug Dependents

1. Knowledge of the patient's level of functioning is necessary to form an appropriate plan of care.

2. Obtain drug history, to determine:
   a. Type of substance used (drug).
   b. Time of last abuse and amount consumed.
   c. Duration and frequency of consumption.
   d. Amount consumed on a daily basis.
3. History from relatives and friends and laboratory investigator to assist drug abuse is essential. Often patient himself may not tell the facts required.
4. Place the patient in a quiet room as excessive stimulation increases patient's agitation.
5. Safety precautions:
   a. Avoid getting drugs from outside sources.
   b. Prevent deliberate self-harm (attempted suicide). Patient's safety is a nursing priority.
6. Medication as instructed by the doctor.

NURSE ROLE IN DRUG ABUSE

- Treating the drug addict
- Hospitalization
- Withdrawal of drugs/detoxification
- Administration of vitamins and pain killers
- Supportive psychotherapy
- Rehabilitation.

Role of Patients

- Love and concern
- Good role model
- Relapse
- Poor follow-up
- Poor rehabilitation services
- Continuous peer pressure.

Prevention

1. Parents—stable home environment.
   Keep child occupied.
   Keep child informed of hazards of drug addiction.
2. Community: At college—misuse of freedom.
   Teacher—teach about hazards of drug addiction.
   Poster—message in society.

3. Legal Control—LAW
   10 years imprisonment and Rupees one lakh fine for possessing and selling and consuming the drugs.
4. Research—statistically prove the status of drug addiction whether increased or decreased.

Medical Intervention for Detoxification as Follows

1. Alcohol.
   Tablet chlordiazepoxide (librium) 40–150 mg in divided doses injection diazepam 10 mg IM/IV, if necessary.
   Multivitamin therapy in combination with daily thiamine injection.
   IV fluids (dextrose). Injection ranitidine/tablet ranitidine and antacid for alcohol induced gastritis.
2. Narcotics (Injections like pentazocine, buprenorphine).
   - Antianxiety/antipsychotic drugs to reduce agitation and restlessness to quieten the patient
   - Non-narcotic analgesics (like ibuprofen)
   - Rest and IV fluids
   - Vitamins
   - Narcotic antagonists, such as naloxone.
3. Cannabis
   - Rest in a quiet place
   - Antianxiety drugs (chlordiazepoxide) to reduce agitation craving and to induce good sleep
   - Good nutritious food
   - Antidepressants or antipsychotics to treat any associated psychiatric complications.

Chapter

17

Organic Mental Disorders Dementia and Delirium

DEFINITION

Organic mental disorders are psychiatric disturbance resulting from transient or permanent central nervous system dysfunction. These are mental illnesses caused by an underlying brain pathology.

All these disorders are associated with transient or permanent dysfunction of the brain. Organic mental disorders are classified as:

1. Acute organic mental disorder (Delirium)
2. Chronic organic mental disorder (Dementia).

The chronic condition (dementia) usually has a somewhat insidious onset. The progression of deterioration is slow and often irreversible. Acute conditions (delirium) have a sudden onset of symptoms. Impairment may usually be reversible with time and treatment.

Comparison of the features of delirium and dementia:

Delirium

Dementia

1. Acute onset
   Insidious onset.
2. Presence of disorientation, anxiety, and poor attention
   Disturbed memory personality deterioration.
3. Clouding of consciousness or drowsiness
   Clear consciousness.
4. Perceptual abnormalities common illusions and hallucinations)
   Global impairment of are cerebral function.

5. Fluctuating course
   Progressive course.
6. Reversible
   Mostly irreversible.

DELIRIUM (ACUTE ORGANIC MENTAL DISORDER)

Delirium is a transient organic mental disorder characterized by generalized physiological dysfunction, usually fluctuating in degree.

Mild delirium is common in general hospital patients.

Clinical Features of Delirium

- Sudden onset
- Prodromal period with insomnia and nightmares
- Clouding of consciousness, drowsiness, restlessness and inattentiveness.
- Disorientation
- Impaired attention span
- Confused, incoherent and unintelligible talk
- Perplexed and fearful mood
- Restlessness and agitation
- Illusion (mostly visual)
- Visual and auditory hallucinations
- Delusional ideas.

Delirium is characterized by a tendency to fluctuate in severity, during the course of the day, i.e. quiet during the day and disturbed at night. The patient cannot remember his disturbed behavior of the previous night (amnesia).

Delirium lasts for a few days to two weeks. Mild delirium is common in the elderly and severely ill patients. Severe delirium is common in severe infectious diseases, alcohol withdrawal and severe metabolic diseases like liver failure and uremia.

Important Causes of Delirium

Infections: Typhoid, pneumonia, septicemia, puerperal sepsis, peritonitis.

Intracranial infections: Encephalitis, meningitis, neurosyphilis cerebral abscess, cerebral malaria.

Acute brain disorders: Head injury, cerebral hemorrhage, hypertensive encephalopathy.

Metabolic disturbance: Uremia, liver failure, cardiac failure, respiratory failure, electrolyte imbalance.

Vitamin deficiency: Pellagra (nicotinamide deficiency), Wernicke's encephalopathy (Thiamine deficiency).

Drug withdrawal: Withdrawal from opiates, barbiturates and alcohol (Delirium tremens).

Drug intoxication: Atropine, cocaine, bromides.

Management of Delirium

1. Identify the likely causes from the patient's history.
2. Investigate and treat the underlying illness with appropriate medical or surgical measures.
3. Correct the symptoms, e.g. hyperpyrexia to be treated, correcting fluid and electrolyte imbalance, giving large doses of vitamin B.
4. Sedation for disturbed patients.

Nursing Care of Delirium

If the patient is agitated, physical restraint may be necessary. Restraint may be preferable to medication if a definite diagnosis has not been made.

Check the Patient's Vital Signs.

Diet: Delirious patients can become exhausted and die, so adequate nourishment and sleep are important. The patient should be gently persuaded to take small meals and frequent drinks of milk, water or fruit juice. Fluid intake should be recorded.

Rest: The patient must be encouraged to rest as much as possible. He will be less confused if he is kept away from noice and activity. The room should be well lit. Shadows and darkness only increase the fear of a confused patient.

Reassurance and Support

The nurse should always remain with a delirious person and must be ready to reassure him in a kindly, soothing voice. The nurse's behavior has great effect upon them and their well-being.

The patient's safety and security is a nursing priority. The nurse should periodically try to orient the patient, i.e. tell him the day, date and time.

Nursing for Delirium

- Nurses should be particularly vigilant in assessing patient who are at Increased risk.
- Assess current and past health status

- Physical examination and review of systems
- Assist for physical functions (activities of daily living)
- Pharmacologic assessments (alcohol and medication)
- Safe and therapeutic environment
- Maintain fluid and electrolyte balance
- Adequate nutrition
- Monitoring and managing side effects
- Encourage to express their fears and discomfort
- Provide support environment with families
- The nurse may encounter patients with delirium in a number of treatment settings, e.g. home, nursing home, ambulatory care, day treatment, outpatient setting and hospital.

DEMENTIA

Dementia (Chronic Organic Mental Disorder)

Dementia is an acquired global impairment of intellect, memory and personality without impairment of consciousness.

Dementia has been identified as a public health problem in recent years. With an increasing number of the elderly, there is a likelihood of increased prevalence of dementia.

Dementia is a syndrome due to disease of the brain, chronic and progressive in nature. There is disturbance of multiple higher cortical functions, including memory, thinking, orientation, comprehension, learning capacity, language and judgment. Consciousness is not disturbed.

Dementia is like a dying mind in a living body: It is not normal ageing or accelerated ageing, but a qualitative and quantitative change in the brain's function. Dementia affects at least 5 percent of the population aged over 65 and 10 percent of those aged over 80.

Classification of Dementia

Senile dementia of Alzheimer's type
Vascular dementia
Dementia in other diseases

- in Pick's disease,
- in Creutzfeldt-Jakob disease
- in Huntington's disease
- in Parkinson's disease
- in HIV disease
- Unspecified dementia.

The Common Causes of Dementia

1. Degenerative (cortical)
   - Alzheimer's disease
   - Pick's disease.
2. Subcortical degenerative
   - Parkinson's disease
   - Huntington's disease
   - Progressive supranuclear palsy
   - 'Punch-drunk' syndrome.
3. Infection and inflammation
   - Neurosyphilis (GPI)
   - AIDS
   - Creutzfeldt-Jakob disease (slow virus)
   - Multiple sclerosis
   - Post-encephalitis.
4. Toxic
   - Alcohol
   - Carbon monoxide
   - Heavy metal poisoning.
5. Metabolic
   - Hypothyroidism
   - Hypocalcemia
   - Hypoglycemia
   - Hepatic encephalopathy
   - Chronic uremia and dialysis
   - Vitamin B12 deficiency
   - Pellagra
6. Tumors
   - Meningioma
   - Benign glioma
   - Para-pituitary tumors
   - Secondary deposits
   - Subdural hematoma
   - Normal pressure hydrocephalus.
7. Trauma
   - Head injury.

Clinical Features of Dementia

Impairment of

1. Memory
2. Thinking and judgment

3. Orientation
4. Comprehension and learning capacity
5. Calculation
6. Language.

Diagnostic Criteria for Dementia

1. Evidence of organic change
2. Evidence of impairment in short- and long-term memory.
3. Impairment in abstract thinking, judgment and higher cortical function and personality change.
4. Disturbance that are interfering with work and social activities.

Alzheimer's dementia is a primary degenerative cerebral disease of unknown etiology. Usually insidious in onset, it develops slowly, but steadily over a period of years. The incidence is higher in later life. Sometimes, the onset may be during presenile period. Alzheimer's dementia is the most common type of dementia in old age. All the features of dementia are present. Diagnostic features are disorientation, memory impairment, poor concentration, poor judgment and slowness in thinking. Brain biopsy shows excessive senile plaques, neurofibrillary tangles and granules and ventricular dilatation.

Multi infarct dementia (vascular dementia): It is caused by chronic anoxia from atherosclerosis. This disorder is associated with cerebral and systemic vascular disease. Commonly, there is accompanying hypertension. The course of the dementia is stepwise and fluctuating. Patchy cognitive disturbances may also be present.

Pick's disease: A dementing condition associated with asymmetric atrophy of the frontal and temporal lobes. It is common in females.

Huntington's chorea: A dementing disease with an autosomal dominant transmission, presenting with insidious onset of involuntary choreiform movement. The average age of onset is in the 30s.

Creutzfeldt-Jakob disease: A rare, rapidly progressing dementia known to be transmitted through a slow acting virus. Death usually occurs in two years.

Normal-pressure hydrocephalus: Occurs mainly in the 7th and 8th decades and may be present with dementia. Unsteadiness of gait, urinary incontinence and nystagmus.

General paralysis of insane (GPI): A condition of neurosyphilis leading on to dementia. Develops usually 10–20 years after initial infection (syphilis). There is atrophy of the cerebral cortex more severe in the frontal and temporal areas. Dementia is associated with depression, mania or schizophreniform psychosis. Other features include epilepsy, Argyll Robertson pupils, tremor, cerebellar or extrapyramidal symptoms, dysarthria, aphasia and hemiplegia.

Management of Dementia

1. Drug treatment: There is no specific drug which can cure dementia, but drugs like hydergine, papaverine, piracetam lecithin are claimed to improve dementia, but associated behavioral problems, psychosis, epilepsy and sleep disturbance can be treated with specific drugs.
2. Psychosocial management
   - Behavioral methods
   - Milieu therapy
   - Activity engagement
   - Physical exercise
   - Problem orientated approach
   - Reality orientation
   - Organization of psychiatric services.

Nursing Care of Dementia

1. Assess patient's level of functioning to formulate appropriate plan of care.
2. Patient's safety is a nursing priority. Assess patient's level of disorientation/confusion to determine specific requirements for safety. Nurse the patient in familiar surroundings, without obstacles.
3. Disorientation may endanger the patient's safety if he unknowingly wanders away from the safe environment. Always instruct the relatives to tie a plastic or aluminium identity tag, so that he can be identified.
4. Dementia patients are prone to aggressive and violent behavior. The nurse should recognize these. Before the patient becomes violent and unmanageable, if necessary, use restraints, but judiciously. Maintain a calm manner with the patient, use drugs as prescribed by the doctors.
5. Use simple explanations and face to face introduction and communication with the patient.
6. Decrease the amount of stimuli in the patient's environment, so that confusion will be less, e.g. low noise level, few people.
7. Provide reassurance if patient is frightened and agitated.
8. Provide feeling of security and stability by allowing the same persons to take care regularly.
9. Help the patient to devise methods to reduce memory defect, e.g. ask them to note down the daily activities and things to be done.
10. Allow the patient to be as independent as possible in self-care activities.
11. Dementia patients may often have problems with elimination (e-g. bed wetting). Measures to educate the patient's relatives to understand the problems of incontinence and to cover the mattress may be taken.

12. Educating the carer (e.g. the relatives) about the gradual decline of mental capacities and the patient's inability to understand the problems they have. The caregiver should understand that the patient becomes dependent and needs support for his activities of daily living.

Nursing Care for Dementia

- Geropsychiatric nursing assessment
- Nursing assessment include medical history, current medical history, and current medication profile
- Physical examination and review of body systems
- Physical functions
- Self care deficit
- Sleep-wake disturbance
- Activity and exercise
- Nutrition
- Chronic pain
- Impaired urinary elimination
- Deficit fluid volume
- Risk for impaired skin integrity
- Ineffective health maintenance and impaired home maintenance
- Impaired memory
- Disturbed thought process
- Chronic confusion
- Disturbed sensory perception
- Impaired environmental interpretation syndrome
- Risk for violence
- Ineffective sexuality patterns
- Ineffective individual coping
- Hopelessness
- Psychiatric aspects of head injury.

Most common causes of head injury are:

1. Road accidents
2. Fall from height
3. Injury associated with alcoholism and quarrels.

During the acute stage of head injury there may be:

1. Loss of consciousness
2. Amnesia-retrograde, post-traumatic
3. Delirium and fits
4. Subdural hematoma.

Psychiatric Complications of Head Injury

1. Dementia.
2. Organic personality syndrome.
3. Schizophrenia like psychosis associated with injuries to temporal lobe.
4. Postconcussion syndrome.
5. Compensation neurosis.

Psychiatric Aspects of Parkinsonism

Parkinsonism is a common and disabling condition, mostly appearing after the age of 50 years. Parkinsonism is an extrapyramidal disorder characterized by:

1. Rigidity.
2. Bradykinesia (slow movement).
3. Tremor at rest.

Causes of Parkinsonism

1. Idiopathic (commonest cause).
2. Infective.
3. Vascular.
4. Metabolic.
5. Toxic.
6. Degenerative.
7. Drug-induced (e.g. antipsychotics).

Drug-induced Parkinsonism is a common picture seen in the psychiatric set-up and antipsychotics like haloperidol, trifluoperazine and chlorpromazine may produce Parkinson features in some patients. The psychiatric problems associated with Parkinsonism are:

1. Dementia.
2. Depression.
3. Psychosis.

Chapter 18

Epilepsy (Seizure Disorder)

INTRODUCTION

Epilepsy is the name given to a sudden loss of consciousness which is often accompanied by repeated jerky movements called convulsions. These attacks are sometimes called fits or seizures. Epilepsy is due to a disturbance in the electrical activity of the brain. It is a condition of cerebral dysrhythmia associated with altered states of consciousness and motor and/or sensory disturbances.

The most characteristic aspects of epilepsy are the repetitiveness and recovery after an attack. It can start at any age. In a majority of the cases, it starts in childhood and adolescence. It is estimated that about 8 to 10 persons in 1000 have this problem at any one time.

CAUSES OF EPILEPSY

Epilepsy, which has no known physical or other cause, is primary or idiopathic epilepsy. It is more common in children and adolescents. When the cause of epileptic fit is known the condition is called secondary or symptomatic epilepsy

Causes

1. Primary epilepsy: Unknown-genetic or biochemical predisposition.
2. Secondary epilepsy:

INTRACRANIAL

- Tumor
- Vascular (infarct or hemorrhage)
- Arteriovenous malformation
- Trauma (birth injury, depressed fracture, penetrating wound)
- Infection (abscess, meningitis, encephalitis)
- Congenital and hereditary disease (tuberous sclerosis).

EXTRACRANIAL

- Metabolic
- Electrolyte
- Biochemical
- Inborn errors of metabolism
- Anoxia
- Hypoglycemia
- Drugs
- Drug withdrawal
- Alcohol withdrawal.

TYPES OF EPILEPSY

There are three types of epilepsy:

1. Grand mal or generalized epilepsy.
2. Focal epilepsy (including temporal lobe epilepsy).
3. Focal epilepsy becoming generalized.

Grand Mal Epilepsy

The attack or fit occurs suddenly and at any place or time. The patient falls down and loses awareness of his surroundings (unconsciousness). This is associated with a loud cry. Face becomes red, eye balls roll up. This is followed by stiffness of the whole body and then by jerky movements of arms, legs and the whole body in a rhythmic manner. At this stage, froth comes out of the mouth. At times, the person urinates in his clothes. Gradually, the jerky movements reduce and the patient becomes completely silent and often goes off to sleep or wakes up as if nothing has happened. This order of events occurring grand mal seizure can be of four stages.

1. Aura.
2. Tonic.
3. Clonic.
4. Recovery.

After an attack, there may be post-epileptic confusion or automatic behavior.

Focal Epilepsy

The convulsions (jerky movements) start in one part of the body like hand or leg or a side of the face. It may be confined to that part only or followed by generalized epilepsy.

Temporal Lobe Epilepsy or Complex Partial Seizure (TLE)

Here, the patient usually does not have a convulsion but enters a dream-like state, and he may have frightening visions or hear strange voices.

Sometimes, he is very confused and may attack other people. When he recovers from the attack he may not remember what has happened. This type of epilepsy is often mistaken for a psychiatric illness.

Status Epilepticus

This is a state of complicated epilepsy. This condition is a psychiatric emergency. Patient gets frequent attacks of fits without regaining consciousness between each attack.

The nurse working in a psychiatric set-up is likely to meet three kinds of problems in relation to epilepsy.

1. The treatment of the psychiatric and social complications of epilepsy
2. The treatment of epilepsy itself.
3. The psychological side-effects of anti-epileptic drugs.

Epilepsy and Mental Illness

A majority of the people who suffer from epilepsy never need to be treated in a psychiatric hospital. However, like other people, epileptics can become mentally ill. Occasionally, an epileptic patient is admitted to a hospital because his behavior is disturbed.

He may become irritable, suspicious or hostile. Sometimes, the chronic epileptics are slow and clumsy in their movements and at times they are confused. Often they find difficulty in putting their thoughts together. Young epileptics often have temper tantrums. Earlier, the textbooks used to describe an epileptic personality type (dependent, rigid, persevering, religious), but many experts now think that this description is only applicable to a few epileptic patients.

Psychiatric Disorders of Seizures

Psychiatric Disorders Directly Related to the Seizures

1. During the preictal (fit) period prodromal symptoms like mood changes, irritable and suspicious behavior can occur.
2. The ictal period, as in TLE has symptoms including autonomic symptoms, mood changes, sensory symptoms, illusions, hallucinations, delusions, forced thinking and memory disturbance

3. The ictal and postictal period has
   a. Psychomotor attacks
   b. Post-epileptic automatism
   c. Confusion and delusion
   d. Twilight state-a dreamy state
   e. Fugue-state of wandering
   f. Violent behavior.

Psychiatric Disorders between Seizures

1. Depression, which may be a reaction to the epileptic illness.
2. Hysterical fits-attention-seeking behavior (hystero epilepsy).
3. A psychosis resembling paranoid schizophrenia (epileptic psychosis)

Chronic Organic Brain Syndrome (dementia) due to Long-term Seizures

Diagnosis

Epilepsy is diagnosed with the help of a reliable and good history. Secondary epilepsies can be identified by investigations like:

- Blood, VDRL, calcium, sugar
- X-ray
- EEG, CT Brain scan, MRI, PET scan.

MANAGEMENT

Drug treatment is useful in controlling epilepsy. In secondary seizures, the primary cause has to be treated. The common anticonvulsants used are:

- Phenytoin sodium
- Carbamazepine
- Sodium valproate
- Diazepam
- Phenobarbitone.

The Nursing Care of Epilepsy

Nursing care during an attack

The nurse should know what she must do and what she must not do during a seizure:

Dos

1. Keep calm. Help the patient lie down, remove glasses, loosen tight clothing.

2. Clear the area of hard, sharp or hot objects which could hurt him. Keep rolled up towel or pillow under his head.
3. Turn him to the side to drain saliva from mouth, which prevent aspiration.
4. After the attack, if the patient is sleepy allow him to rest.

Don'ts

1. Do not allow people to gather around him. Allow free air circulation and open all windows.
2. Do not restrain the convulsive movements (fit).
3. Do not force anything between his tightly held teeth.
4. Do not offer anything to eat or drink till he is fully conscious.

You Have to Call a Doctor

- If patient is injured
- Has repeated seizures?
- Is unconscious for a long time?
- Has difficulty in breathing?
- If it is going to be the first attack, especially after the age of 40.

Nursing Care of Status Epilepticus

Status epilepticus is an emergency condition. The nurse should inform the doctor at once. Meanwhile, she has to start oxygen and intravenous fluids. Injection diazepam 10 mg slow intravenous is the treatment of choice.

Long-term Nursing Care of Epileptic Patients

Health education regarding epilepsy to the patient's relatives to the community is very essential. Misconceptions about epilepsy are to be clarified. The nurse should educate them of the following important facts:

1. Epilepsy is not due to sin or evil spirits—it is a disease due to disturbances in the brain function.
2. Epilepsy can be effectively cured. Medical treatment is essential and should be started during the initial stage itself.
3. Long-term maintenance of drug treatment is essential for complete cure. Treatment should be continued till the patient is fit free for a three year period. Then, after consultation with the doctor, the treatment can be stopped.
4. Few patients require continued treatment to control their fits. It is only for very few patients that drug treatment may not respond.

5. Patients and relatives should be educated to identify certain side effects of drugs given for treatment. Some of the side effects are unsteadiness of gait, slurring of speech, double vision, etc. This has to be immediately brought to the notice of the doctor.
6. Hot water baths, frequent watching of television and sudden exposure to powerful lights may precipitate an attack.
7. Patients suffering from epilepsy can have normal marital life.
8. They can be employed anywhere except those places involving heavy machinery, fire and driving.

Chapter 19

Mental Retardation

Mental Retardation is below average general intellectual functioning originating during the development period and associated with impairment in adaptive behavior.

Mental retardation (MR) is a condition of arrested or incomplete development of the mind. It is a subnormal state of intelligence. Mental retardation is not an illness, but a condition of poor development of the brain. Mental retardation is otherwise known as mental subnormality or mental deficiency or mentally handicap.

Mental retardation can occur any time before eighteen years of age. Some degree of mental retardation is seen in 1 to 2 percent of the general population. Growth and development is slow in mentally retarded children. Mentally retarded children can have associated conditions like fits, hearing, visual or physical handicap or behavioral problems.

Normally a child of certain physical or chronological age should have a mental age that corresponds to the physical age. When the mental age is lesser than the physical age, such a child is considered mentally retarded. Intelligence of a person is referred to in terms of intelligence quotient (IQ). It is calculated from mental age (MA) and chronological age (CA) as follows:

$$IQ = \frac{\text{Mental age} \times 100}{\text{Chronical age}}$$

If the IQ is less than 70 it is considered to be mental retardation.

CLASSIFICATION

Mental retardation is classified on the basis of IQ as follows:

Levels	IQ range
1. Mild mental retardation	50–69
2. Moderate mental retardation	35–49
3. Severe mental retardation	20–34
4. Profound mental retardation	Below 20

Based on practical applications mental retardation can be classified into three groups:

1. Educable group.
2. Trainable group.
3. Custodial group.

RECOGNITION OF MENTAL RETARDATION IN CHILDREN

Mental retardation can be recognized in the following ways:

1. By talking to the parents, especially mother, in detail about the growth of the child.
2. By observing the child's physical appearance and behavior.

Mental retardation can be recognized from a history of delayed developmental milestones. Following are the important normal milestones of development.

3 months—Holding neck erect
6 months—Sitting with support
9 months—One year walking
1½ years—Speaking few words or phrases.

Mental retardation can be identified at different stages of growth through the following ways.

1. Below five years—Through history of delayed milestones.
2. Above five years—Through history of school failures, behavior problems and behavior against society's expectations.

PHYSICAL APPEARANCE

Mentally retarded children have certain physical features which make them easily identifiable. These features are common in the severely retarded. Some mild and moderate retarded children do not have any physical abnormalities and look normal. The common abnormalities seen in mental retardation are:

- Small (or) large head
- Slanting eyes
- Thick protruding tongue
- Microcephaly, hydrocephalus
- Rough skin
- Stunted growth.

CAUSES OF MENTAL RETARDATION

Genetic

Chromosome abnormalities

- Down's syndrome
- Klinefelter's syndrome
- Turner's syndrome.

Metabolic Disorders Affecting

- Amino acids (e.g. phenylketonuria, homocystinuria, Hartnup disease)
- The urea cycle (e.g. citrullinuria, aminosuccinic aciduria)
- Lipids (Tay-Sachs, Gaucher's and Niemann-Pick diseases
- Carbohydrate (Lesch-Nyhan syndrome)
- Mucopolysaccharidoses (Hurler's, Hunter's, Sanfilippo; Morquio's syndrome).

Gross Disease of the Brain

- Tuberous sclerosis
- Neurofibromatosis.

Cranial Malformations

- Hydrocephalus
- Microcephalus.

Antenatal Damage

- Infections (rubella, cytomegalo virus, syphilis, toxoplasmosis, AIDS)
- Intoxications (lead, certain drugs, alcohol)
- Physical damage (injury, radiation, hypoxia)
- Placental dysfunction (toxemia, nutritional growth retardation
- Endocrine disorders (hypothyroidism, hypoparathyroidism).

Perinatal

- Birth asphyxia
- Complications of prematurity
- Kernicterus
- Intraventricular hemorrhage.

Postnatal Damage

- Injury (accidental, child abuse)
- Lead intoxication
- Infection (encephalitis, meningitis)
- Malnutrition.

COMMON CAUSES OF MENTAL RETARDATION IN OUR COUNTRY

1. Infection during infancy—Encephalitis meningitis.
2. During pregnancy—rubella, syphilis, AIDS, etc.
3. Nutritional deficiency during pregnancy and childhood.
4. Primary and genetically related causes.
5. Chromosomal abnormality, e.g. Down's syndrome.
6. Endocrine-Cretinism due to hypothyroidism.
7. Phenylketonuria-biochemical abnormality.

Down's Syndrome

A condition of mental retardation caused by a chromosomal abnormality. Down's syndrome children usually have trisomy in 21st chromosome (instead of usual pair, there are 3 chromosomes).

The features of Down's syndrome include stunted growth, oblique palpebral fissure, small flattened head, high cheek bones, big mouth and small fingers. They are moderate-to-severely mentally retarded. They are cheerful and lovable children,

Cretinism

A mentally retarded condition due to hypothyroidism. Symptoms begin to appear around the age of six months.

Clinical features include stunted physical growth, grayish-yellowish color of the skin, puffy face, reduced pulse rate, subnormal temperature, slow (usually) and retarded activity, apathy and lethargy. They are of moderate-to-severely mentally retarded.

Treatment: Oral thyroid preparation (thyroxine). If treatment is started very early the prognosis is good.

Phenylketonuria

A condition of mental retardation due to an inborn error of metabolism. This is an autosomal recessive disorder. The metabolism of the essential amino acid phenylalanine is disturbed. There is an inability to convert phenylalanine to tyrosine. This is due to the absence or inactiveness of an enzyme known as phenylalanine hydroxylase.

Treatment: Phenylalanine—free diet from very early infancy.

REHABILITATION AND NURSING CARE OF THE MENTALLY RETARDED

Rehabilitation depends upon their disability. It can be assessed through IQ and clinical evaluation. It must be remembered that there are three aspects to the problem of the mentally retarded.

1. The impairment itself. For example, brain injury as a result of prenatal or infection.
2. The disability which results, e.g. inability to read or to perform arithmetic.
3. The social handicap in which the disability results. For example, resultant problem with regard to occupation, or personal relationships.

Assessment of the need: As soon as mental retardation is suspected, it is essential to assess whether the condition is treatable and reversible. Then, it is important to assess whether the person can be educated and trained (if the mental retardation is mild and moderate) or, if custodial care only is possible (if the mental retardation is severe and profound).

Education of Mentally Retarded Children

Mild and moderate mentally retarded children can have a planned education program in a special school meant for these children. Here, these children will be helped by specially trained teachers to read, write and develop to the best of their ability. Mentally retarded children require early stimulation. Parents of mentally retarded children have an important role in this regard, but require guidance from trained personnel.

Training the Mentally Retarded

Mild and moderate mentally retarded persons require special training, if possible, in sheltered workshops, under supervision, to acquire skills in simple jobs like gardening, book binding, paper cover making, etc. They require training by specially trained teachers or occupational therapists. To learn simple tasks they may require much longer time than normal children, hence, much patience is required to train them. The purpose of this occupation is to give the mentally retarded a meaningful and useful life, so that he should not depend on others for their daily needs.

Custodial Care of the Mentally Retarded

Some severe or profound mentally retarded require custodial care either at home or in the institutions like special centers or mental hospitals.

The indications for institutional care include:

1. Severely mentally retarded without any social support.
2. Severely mentally retarded with behavioral problems.
3. Severe mental retardation with complications like intractable epilepsy.
4. Institutionalization for short time for the convenience of the family members, e.g. during the time of some functions at home.

Some severely mentally retarded children are so physically disabled that they have to be nursed in bed. In such cases, specialized nursing is the most important part of treatment. For every physical need, they require assistance. The nursing care includes training to walk, toilet training ,and training to eat properly.

As the years go, these mentally retarded children will gradually learn things, but very slowly.

PREVENTION OF MENTAL RETARDATION

Mental retardation can be prevented in the following ways:

Before Conceiving (for mothers)

- Rubella immunization
- Genetic counseling
- Health education for pregnant mothers including advice about nutritious diet, avoiding smoking and drinking alcohol
- Use of contraception and family planning methods to avoid unwanted pregnancies
- As much as possible to avoid consanguineous marriages.

Prenatal

- Identification of risk groups and genetic counseling
- Rubella screening
- Syphilis and AIDS screening
- Diagnostic ultrasound of growth retardation
  - Microcephalus
  - Hydrocephalus
  - Multiple births
- Improved antenatal care with special reference to factors leading to low birth weight.

Natal

Improved obstetric and neonatal care (with the aim of reducing hypoxia and birth trauma).

Postnatal

- Neonatal screening of treatment of hypothyroidism and phenyl-ketonuria
- Prompt surgical treatment of hydrocephalus
- Improved care on immunization to reduce incidence of encephalitis and meningitis
- Prevention of further damage of impaired children, e.g. control of epilepsy
- Preventive measures to reduce child abuse, road traffic accidents and home accidents.

HEALTH EDUCATION REGARDING MENTAL RETARDATION

As far as possible, the mentally retarded children should be taken care of at home, so that they get emotional support.

- Mental retardation cannot be cured, but can be improved through proper care
- Mentally retarded children improve with training, but slowly
- Mentally retarded children require:
  - Good food
  - Love and affection
  - Special education and training
  - Good social support.
- Mental retardation is due to poor development of the brain. The two to three out of a hundred children are to some extent, retarded. It is a medical problem and not due to fate, one's misdeeds or bad luck
- Medicines cannot cure mental retardation, but complications such as behavioral problems and epilepsy can be effectively controlled by them
- The goal of rehabilitation of the mentally retarded is to make them as independent as possible
- Marriage is not a cure for mental retardation. Moderate-to-severely retarded persons cannot take the responsibilities of marital life.

Parent's Counseling

The parents of mentally retarded children require life-long adjustment. Hence, the parents need guidance and counseling which is an important aspect of the management of the mentally retarded. This will help the parents to understand and to accept the child's problems and in making plans according to the capacity of the mentally retarded person.

Counseling should focus on:

a. Giving information regarding the condition of the mentally retarded child.
b. Developing the right attitude towards the handicapped child.
c. Educating the parents regarding their role in the training of the retarded child.

The parents should:

1. Understand the actual condition of the mentally retarded child.
2. Not harbor false hopes regarding cure or improvement.
3. Have available information regarding professional help for treating associated conditions or complications like seizures (epilepsy), hyperactivity and psychosis.
4. Avoid attitudes like rejection or overprotection.
5. Not feel guilty, depressed or responsible for the condition.

Their cooperation and support is essential in the rehabilitation of the mentally retarded.

- Nursing consideration
- Management
- Skill training
- Behavior modification
- Parent counseling
- Prevention
- Prenatal
- Perinatal
- Postnatal.

NURSING MANAGEMENT

- Accurate observation and recording of behavior and skills present
- Nutritional requirement
- Elimination needs
- Maintenance of hygiene
- Communication need
- Assisting in skill training and behavior modification program
- Parent education and guidance in skill training.

SKILL TRAINING

- Develop mental skills
- Self care skills

- Communication skills
- Home living skills
- Community skills
- Self direction skills
- Healthy and safety skills
- Work skills.

Training activities to be divided into small steps, demonstrated repeatedly, regularly, and systematically.

BEHAVIOR MODIFICATION

a. For decreasing undesirable behavior restructure environment.
   Extinction
   Punishment (Time out, aversion, restraint, etc.)
b. For increasing desirable behavior token program
   Shaping
   Chaining, generalization, imitation, cueing
3. Parent counseling.

STAGE

I: Impart information regarding condition
II: Create awareness regarding role in training the child
III: Develop right attitudes by correcting misconceptions.

Chapter

20

Other Disorders

SEXUAL DISORDERS

It is difficult to define what is normal or abnormal in sexual behavior. Patterns of morality, social norms and customs vary in different countries and cultures as well as change over short periods of time. The term abnormal, consequently tends to mean unusual rather than pathological.

Normal sexual behavior usually means any activity, which an heterosexual relationship leads to intercourse and orgasm.

The important aspects of normal sexual behavior are:

1. Sex drive: This motivates the person to seek sexual stimulation. It is a strong driving force in determining human behavior.
2. Sexual arousal: Sexual arousal is a response to sexual stimulation. Different people are aroused by different stimuli which include sights, sounds, smell, touch and fantasy.
3. Genital response: This is a response to sexual arousal. In the male, the genital response is rapid. The essential component is penile erection. In the female, the genital response is slow. The essential components are vasocongestion of the vulva and labia minora and vaginal secretion. The genital response is accompanied by increase in blood pressure and heart rate.
4. Orgasm: In the male, it is a pleasurable experience accompanied by ejaculation or forceful expulsion of semen from the urethra. In the female, it a pleasurable experience accompanied by a spasm of the muscles of the outer third of the vagina.

Psychosexual disorders can be grouped under the following headings:

1. Sexual dysfunction not caused by organic disorder (sexual inadequacies).
2. Gender identity disorder or transsexualism.
3. Disorders of sexual preference
   - Fetishism
   - Transvestism
   - Exhibitionism

- Voyeurism
- Pedophilia
- Sadism
- Masochism.

4. Sexual orientation disorder—homosexuality
   Sexual Inadequacies.

Common sexual inadequacies are:
In the male:

1. Erectile impotence—inability to sustain an erection adequate for penetration.
2. Premature ejaculation—ejaculation before, during or immediately after penetration.

In the female

1. Frigidity—Orgasm rarely or never achieved.
2. Vaginismus—Involuntary contraction of vaginal introitus at penetration.

In India, females rarely complain about sexual inadequacies. The most common complaint is male erectile impotence.

Erectile Impotence (Impotence)

It is the inability to reach an erection or sustain it longer enough for satisfactory penetration. Only when it affects 75 percent of the sexual attempts it is considered a disorder. It may be accompanied by premature ejaculation.

Causes of impotence

1. Medical Illness
   - Diabetes mellitus, thyroid disorder
     - Testicular atrophy
     - Hypertension
   - Genital abnormalities
     - Spinal cord lesions
     - Brain damage.
2. Psychiatric disorders
   - Anxiety, drug dependence
   - Schizophrenia
   - Alcoholism and depression.
3. Drugs that may produce impotence
   - Antihypertensive drugs like propranolol, methyldopa, clonidine
   - Hormonal preparations—steroids, estrogen
   - Anticholinergic drugs

- Psychotropic drugs, antipsychotic drugs
- Some antidepressants
- Anti-inflammatory drugs like indomethacin.

4. Psychosocial factors
   - Performance anxiety—during early period of marriage situations—lack of privacy, fear of STD or AIDS, fatigue, in-cooperative partner
   - Poor marital relationship
   - Reduced sex drive—old age, ill health
   - Homosexuality.

Management: Rule out medical or psychiatric disorder that may produce impotence.

- Analyze the problems and decide sexual therapy
- Counseling and educating the persons on sexual anatomy, sexual response and sexual practices
- Teach the patient to relieve anxiety through relaxation techniques
- Use some principles of Masters and Johnson's sensate focus technique, in which the couple is to start slowly with no genital stimulation for a few weeks, followed by manual genital stimulation, before, proceeding to attempt sexual intercourse. This reduces anxiety, increases feeling of security and improves communication and understanding.

Gender Identity Disorder—Transsexualism

Transsexualism is a gender identity disorder characterized by a sense of discomfort and a wish to physically become a member of the opposite sex. The patient is psychologically a member of the opposite sex, e.g. a male transsexual believes the he is a woman and he wants to convert himself into a woman by a sex change operation.

Disorders of Sexual Preference

Fetichism: A psychosexual disorder in which sexual arousal and gratification are brought about by objects such as shoes, underwear or toilet articles.

Transvestism: A psychosexual disorder characterized by recurrent and persistent cross-dressing for the purpose of achieving sexual excitement.

Exhibitionism: A psychosexual disorder in which the preferred method of sexual stimulation and gratification consists of repetitive acts of exposing the genitals to strangers.

Voyeurism: A psychosexual disorder in which the preferred method of sexual gratification consists of repetitive observation of people in different states of undress or sexual activity.

Pedophilia: A psychosexual disorder in which the preferred method of sexual stimulation and gratification consists of repetitive sexual activity with children.

Sexual sadism: A psychosexual disorder in which an individual inflicts physical or psychological pain on another person to achieve sexual excitement.

Sexual masochism: A psychosexual disorder in which an individual seeks physical or psychological pain, including humiliation or being bound or beaten, to achieve sexual excitement.

Sexual Orientation Disorder—Homosexuality

Homosexuality is sexual attraction to, and sexual activity with members of the same sex. It usually refers to the male. For females, it is called lesbianism. In India, homosexual activity is an offence. According to an important study, 4 percent of males and 4 percent of single females are homosexual. Their practices vary and they may engage in perverted practices.

Treatment: Most homosexuals do not seek treatment. If they come for psychiatric help they may be benefited by behavior modification therapy.

NURSING CARE FOR SEXUAL DISORDER

Sexual role conflicts

Behaviors of avoidance, withdrawal, and ambiguity
Depression associated with feelings of uselessness
Fears of being seen as emotionally distant or cold.

Somatic complaints

Explore feelings about current and past life situations
Describe realistic ideas about strengths and limitations
Practice assertive communication skill
Determine role behaviors, appropriate to marriage and profession.

SLEEP DISORDERS

Sleep and dreams have been subjects of interest for long years. Sleep can be regarded as a physiological, reversible reduction of conscious awareness. There are two types of sleep:

1. REM sleep (Rapid eye movement sleep)
2. NREM sleep (Non-REM sleep).

REM Sleep is Active Sleep

Characteristics of REM Sleep

- Rapid eye movements
- Dreaming
- Increased brain metabolism
- Oxygen utilization and temperature
- A loss of muscle tone
- Tachycardia
- Arrhythmia, and
- Penile erection.

Characteristics of NREM Sleep

NREM sleep is divided according to its EEG recordings into four stages. NREM sleep is accompanied by a slowdown of bodily functions. There is reduction in heart rate, respiration, urine output, blood pressure, temperature and a state of relaxation in metabolism and motor activities.

Sleep Requirement

Most people require between 6–9 hours of sleep per day. Those who require less than 6 hours of sleep are called 'short sleepers' and those who require more than 9 hours of sleep are called 'long sleepers.'

REM sleep is longer in long sleepers. Short sleepers are generally healthier, active and better adjusted. Sleep requirements increase in children and old people. More hours of sleep are needed in pregnancy, sickness, mental stress, depressed mood and after strenuous work.

Sleep Deprivation

Sleep deprivation is a pressing health problem. If a person is not sleeping continuously for few days or nights, it is harmful to his health.

Sleep Deprivation May Produce

1. Impaired mental alertness and performance.
2. Thinking process is disturbed.
3. Results in poor attention, concentration and judgment.
4. Mental fatigue may even trigger physical illness like heart attack.
5. May lead on to traffic accidents and industrial mishaps.
6. May lead to poor performance in studies and problems like drug abuse in students.

CLASSIFICATION OF SLEEP DISORDERS

Primary sleep disorders (Disordered sleep is the only sign and symptom of abnormality)

a. Cataplexy: Sudden decrease or loss of (sleep paralysis) muscle tone, often generalized and may lead on to sleep.
b. Hypersomnia: Excessive sleep at night or during the day.
c. Insomnia: Inability to fall asleep and maintain sleep. When occurs in the absence of physical or psychological disorders, it is primary insomnia.
d. Kleine-Levin syndrome: Periodic episodes of hypersomnia.
e. Narcolepsy: Uncontrollable, recurrent brief episodes of sleep associated with cataplexy.
f. Nightmares: Sleep disturbance with frightening or bad dreams. A good recall of dream occurs during REM sleep.
g. Night terrors: Sleep disturbance accompanied by panic, confusion and no recall of the frightening dream.
h. Pickwickian: Occurs during stage 4 (NREM) sleep with hypersomnia associated with obesity and respiratory disturbance.

Secondary sleep disorders (Clinical problem accompanied by specific or non-specific disturbances)

a. Alcoholism—Variable sleep disturbance.
b. Anorexia nervosa—Decreased total sleep time.
c. Depression—Less sleep time, more awakenings.
d. Hyperthyroidism—Insomnia.
e. Hypothyroidism—Increased sleep.
f. Schizophrenia—Variable.

Parasomnias (Waking up during sleep)

a. Bruxism (teeth grinding): Occurs during stage 2 (NREM) sleep with loud noise and damage to teeth.
b. Enuresis: Bed wetting during sleep.
c. Sleep talking: Mainly occurs during NREM sleep. Very common by itself or as a part of some other sleep disorder or psychiatric disorders.
d. Sleep walking: Occurs during stage 4 (NREM) sleep, in which, walking or other motor acts are performed.

NURSING CARE IN SLEEP DISORDER

Assess the client's current sleep pattern and take a complete sleep history.

Identify both internal and external factors that are inhibiting the clients sleep.

Ascertain the client's sleep-related routines and rituals. Encourage the client to use sleep-promoting methods.

Encourage the client to maintain a sleep diary or chart and to make a practice of using sleep strategies

Provide comfort measures such as backrubs, comfortable night clothes and prescribed pain medications.

INSOMNIA

Insomnia is defined as quantitatively or qualitatively insufficient sleep on the basis of the individual need. Insomnia is the term applied collectively to complaints involving the chronic inability to obtain adequate sleep. Insomnia is difficulty in falling asleep, difficulty in maintaining sleep or insufficient sleep. Insomnia is of three types.

1. Sleep onset insomnia—difficulty in falling asleep.
2. Frequent noctural awakening—interrupted sleep characterized by frequent awakening.
3. Early morning awakening—waking up early in the morning and not being able to fall back asleep.

Causes of Insomnia

1. Primary—Due to specific sleep disorders.
2. Secondary—Due to
   - Physical causes
   - Behavioral causes
   - Psychiatric disturbances
   - Social causes
   - Drug-related causes.

Physical Causes

Uneasiness, discomfort: Dyspnea, cough, itching, nocturia.
Chronic pains: Headache, neuralgia, cramps, orthopedic disorders, cancer.
Endocrine disorders: Menopause, hyperthyroidism, hypoglycemia.

Behavioral Causes

Naps (during the day)

- Irregular sleeping hours
- Lack of physical exercise
- Alcohol or tobacco abuse
- Excessive coffee in the evening
- Disturbing bed partner
- Disturbing environment (heat, cold, noise).

Psychiatric Disorders

- Depression
- Anxiety
- Hypomania
- Schizophrenia
- Chronic alcoholism and drug addiction.

Social Causes

- Separation or divorce
- Overwork, career change
- Traumatic experience (accident, assault)
- Immigration
- Serious illness in the family
- Birth in the family
- Death of spouse or close relative
- Financial loss
- Acquiring a physical handicap
- Son or daughter leaving home
- Retirement
- Failure (Exam, love).

Drug-Related Causes

- Stimulants
- Thyroid hormones
- Sympathomimetic
- Diuretics
- Corticosteroids
- Beta-blockers.

Treatment of Insomnia

- Detailed assessment and evaluation
- Identifying the causative factors and treating them.

Most of the patients who seek treatment for insomnia suffer from anxiety and depression. Other causes are less common.

Treatment of insomnia depends on duration. Transient insomnia can be treated initially with hypnotics (like nitrazepam, lorazepam, etc.). Hypnotics should not be given for longer-periods.

Non-Drug Treatment for Insomnia

Progressive relaxation: Relax the body (muscle), thereby relaxing the mind.

Autogenic training: Autosuggestion.

Meditation, yoga: Produces relaxation of the mind.

Biofeedback: Self monitoring, keeping record of sleep and walking.

Stimulus control therapy: Do not use the bed for reading or chatting. Go to bed for sleeping only.

Nursing Care of Persons with Insomnia

The common complaint a nurse receives during her night duty is disturbance in sleep. Hence, a nurse should understand in detail, the concept of sleep, the effects of sleep deprivation and various causes of insomnia. Apart from giving medication as prescribed by the doctors, the nurse should be in a position to educate the patient in getting good sleep.

Sleep hygiene: Nurse should advise her patients to avoid heavy meals or exercise before sleep. Coffee, tea or smoking should also be avoided before sleep. Try to minimize the use of hypnotics substitute back rubs, warm milk and relaxation exercises.

Sleep environment: Make the environment conducive to sleep. Too much light, noise and heat or cold are to be avoided. Close doors, dim lights, and turn of unnecessary machinery. Encourage staff to talk in low tones during the night in the wards. The nurse should keep a daily record of how many hours the patient has slept. If there is any sleep disturbance or sleep associated problem, inform the doctor.

MEMORY DISORDERS

Memory is a function by which information stored in the brain is later recalled to consciousness.

There are three processes occurring in memory

1. Registration
2. Retention
3. Recall.

Memory function is generally divided into three categories:

1. Immediate
2. Recent
3. Remote.

Immediate memory: Immediate memory is tested by recalling given digits. The patient is given a series of random numbers (e.g. 2-6-9 or 4-7-5-8} and asked to recall them immediately. Normal persons can repeat an average of six to seven digits forward and four or five digits backward.

Recent memory: Ask the patient how they spent the last 24 hours and what they ate for breakfast.

Remote memory: Ask the patient the important names and dates from his or her earlier life (e.g. birth, marriage, school, jobs).

Disturbances of memory can be classified as follows:

1. Amnesia
2. Paramnesia
   - False recognition
   - Retrospective falsification
   - Confabulation (filling up memory gaps)
   - Dejavu (feeling of familiarity to unknown things or situations)
3. Hypermnesia-Jamais VU (known persons or places look unfamiliar).

NURSING CARE METHODS TO IMPROVE MEMORY

- Select one time and one place for studying
- Keep yourself fresh and the environment pleasant
- Love and keep your motivation high
- Take easily digestible food at regular intervals
- Keep your body fit by regular exercise
- Good study habits.

AMNESIA

Amnesia is loss of memory and partial or total inability to recall past experiences. Amnesia may be anterograde or retrograde.

Anterograde: Amnesia is the inability to recall events occurring after the amnesia causing incident (e.g. head injury or administration of a drug).

Retrograde Amnesia: It is the loss of memory for events that occurred prior to the amnesia causing incident.

Classification of Amnesia

1. Psychogenic
   a. Fugue
   b. Dual and multiple personalities
   c. Ganser state
   d. Slips of the tongue and amnesia for word finding.

2. Organic:
   a. Cerebral disease
   b. Transient global amnesia
   c. Amnestic syndrome
   d. Traumatic amnesia
   e. Temporal lobe amnesia
   f. Amnesia associated with ECT.

Psychogenic Amnesia

Emotional factors produce amnesia and usually affect only the ability to recall experiences. Registration and retention are unaffected.

Psychogenic amnesia is either dense and global or restricted to certain specific themes.

The psychoanalytic theory of psychogenic amnesia is 'forgetting of disagreeable'

Fugue state: A state of amnesia in which the person wanders away from his normal surroundings and is associated with loss of personal identity. Fugue state can occur in hysteria, depression, alcoholism, epilepsy and head injury.

Organic Amnesia

Amnesia in cerebral disease may be transient or persistent.

Transient amnesia states can occur in toxic or metabolic disturbances, due to certain drugs, cerebral anoxia and carbon monoxide, intracranial infection, epilepsy and acute alcoholic intoxication.

Persistent abnormalities of memory can occur in chronic alcoholism, vascular disorders, cerebral tumors, brain operations, dementia, etc.

Confabulation is a memory disturbance commonly seen in alcoholics. Confabulation is a condition of inventing stories about situations or events that are not remembered. It is a condition of filling up of memory.

Transient global amnesia is an organic memory disturbance of acute onset occurring usually in middle age and lasts for four to twelve hours and remits spontaneously. The characteristics are, total loss of memory, confusion, repeated purposeless behavior and some degree of clouding of consciousness, The cause lies within in the temporal lobe.

Amnestic syndrome is an impaired memory state occurring in a state of clear awareness. It may be due to head trauma, hypoxia, thiamine deficiency or encephalitis.

ECT-induced amnesia occurs after electroconvulsive therapy. There is always a transient memory loss. The amnesia is both retrograde and anterograde in nature. The ECT induced amnesia may persist for few weeks and remit spontaneously. Unipolar ECT (keeping the ECT electrodes only on the non-dominant side) and brief pulse ECT may reduce this memory disturbance.

Nursing Care of Amnesia

The nurse should first understand the disturbance of memory is a common symptom in the psychiatric setup. It may be due to psychological or organic factors. Because of amnesia, patient may often not be in a position to give correct history. Hence, it should be cross-checked with relatives later. In short-term memory, disturbances other practical problems may come up. The patient has already had his medication may ask for the drugs again. This specially occurs in the elderly. Medication given should be carefully recorded otherwise a double dose may be given which can have adverse effects. Patients with confabulation give immediate answers. Even though, they seem correct they may be totally false. This should be kept in mind.

EATING DISORDERS

Eating disorders have become the focus of much interest among mental health professionals in recent years. In India, eating disorders are not as common as in the West. An increasing number of people, predominantly women, report gross disturbances in their eating behavior. The two most important eating disorders are:

1. Anorexia nervosa
2. Bulimia.

Although, these eating disorders are described as primary, i.e. as not resulting from some medical illness, many patients with these disorders also suffer from other psychiatric disorders.

ANOREXIA NERVOSA

It is condition of marked weight loss due to reduction in food intake and/or vomiting. The anorexia nervosa syndrome may be secondary to schizophrenia, depression, organic illness and endocrine disorders.

Anorexia nervosa is more common in females, more so in adolescent girls. It is common in the upper social class and in unhappy families. The precipitating events may be separation, puberty, sexual experience, threat of sex, marriage, pregnancy responsibility, etc.

Clinical Picture

The patient is usually an adolescent or young adult female. There may be a history of reduction in the intake of high calorie food and of vomiting.

The other features are amenorrhea, constipation and hyperactivity. The examination shows a low BP, low pulse rate, subnormal temperature, cyanosis, atrophy of breast, axillary and pubic hair. Investigations reveal anemia, low blood sugar, raised cholesterol and reduced basal metabolic rate.

Anorexic nervosa is a potentiality lethal disorder. It should be treated as a psychiatric emergency. If there is severe weight loss, metabolic disturbances, anemia, hypoglycemia and depression with suicidal ideas, the patient should be immediately hospitalized for further management.

Treatment

Treatment includes hospitalization, tube feeding and IV fluid; high calorie diet should be prescribed, drugs like minimal dose chlorpromazine, cyproheptadine and insulin may be beneficial.

Behavior therapy is of much beneficial.

Nursing Care of Anorexia Nervosa

When a nurse sees people, especially young girls, who have eating disorder problem, with poor intake, vomiting, self starvation, severe weight loss, it should be immediately reported.

- Monitor physiologic signs and symptoms like amenorrhea, constipation, hypoglycemia, anemia, breast atrophy, hypotension, etc.
- Weigh regularly
- Have one-to-one supervision during and 30 minutes after meal time to prevent attempts to vomit food
- Health education should be given regarding maintaining normal weight, normal sexual growth and complications of starvation.

BULIMIA

Bulimia is an eating disorder manifested by excessive hunger, resulting in compulsive or overeating. Bulimics lose control over eating behavior and consume large quantities of calorie rich food. Associated with bulimia are other conditions like abuse of alcohol and drugs, laxative abuse, diuretic abuse.

Bulimia nervosa is an eating disorder of unknown etiology occurring in women. Bulimia is often associated with depressed mood and suicidal ideas. Antidepressants, especially tricyclic antidepressants may be beneficial.

Nursing Care for Eating Disorders

- Develop ability to form trust and verbalize feelings by first establishing nurse-patient relationships
- Show appropriate eating pattern
- Weight should be stabilized
- Behavior demonstrating sense of self control
- Involvement in social activities and peer relationship
- Regular balanced sleeping, eating and exercise pattern
- Demonstrate interest in studies and other daily activities
- Realistic perception of body image.

Chapter

21

Mental Health Problems

CHILD/ADOLESCENT/WOMEN/OLD AGE

Children's health has been recognized as an important component of any Nation's health. The concept of good mental health in children has also gained importance in the recent past. Children constitute about 40% of our population.

The mental health problems in children are different from adults, because of the following reasons:

1. The child is a growing organism. Children are in a constant state of rapid physical, emotional and intellectual development. Their personality is not yet fully formed.
2. They are unable to verbalize or express themselves and their problems.
3. They are dependent on their family members, especially parents.
4. They mimic what they observe.

Child psychiatric problems are widely prevalent in India. Figures from various studies in India suggest that 2.5–17.2% of children suffer from some kind of mental health problem.

The commonest psychiatric disorders among children in India are mental retardation, neurotic, psychosomatic disorders and attention deficit disorders. Problems like enuresis and speech disorders, less commonly, conduct disorders.

The causes of child psychiatric disorders are:

1. Biological factors
   - Heredity
   - Physical defects
   - Illness
   - Low intelligence.
2. Psychological factors
   - Parent-child relationship
   - Quarrels between parents
   - Broken homes
   - Discipline
   - Too much discipline
   - Alcoholic father.

3. Social factors
   - Poverty
   - Unhealthy environment.

FAMILY AND CHILD MENTAL HEALTH PROBLEMS

The child's behavior and emotional problems are usually the refraction of the family. "The Child is the biopsy of the family". A healthy child will come only from a happy family. Families are miniature societies in which children learn adaptation and social behavior.

The family should facilitate development, from infantile dependence to adult dependence. Children who are deprived of a happy family life suffer from serious mental health problems at a later date. Parental deprivation, especially maternal deprivation, may be the cause for psychological problems, especially depression in later years. In children, much of the behavioral disorders and personality deviance can be linked to the faulty parental attitudes. Rejection, hostility, and neglect by the parents may damage their psychological equilibrium. In the same way over-protection also will harm the child's mental health.

COMMON MENTAL HEALTH PROBLEMS IN CHILDREN

Mental Retardation and Associated Problems (Discussed in a Different Chapter)

Autistic Disorder

Autistic disorders are characterized by a withdrawal of the child into the self and into a fantasy world of his own creation. This disorder is rare. Course is chronic. It is also known as Infantile Autism, if the age of onset is before three years.

The common symptoms are:

- Failure to form interpersonal relationships
- Impairment in communication
- Bizarre responses to the environment
- Extreme fascination for objects that move (e.g. fans, trains)
- Fluctuating mood-sudden crying or laughing
- Self-mutilative behavior.

Attention Deficit Disorders (Hyperactive disorders)

A disorder occurring in childhood characterized by poor attention span, overactivity and impulsiveness. The child responds to multiple stimuli at the same time.

The common symptoms are:
- Easily distracted; nor able to sit or do one thing for some time.

Disorganized behavior

- Sustaining attention is difficult. Hence is disruptive and overactive in the class room.
- The child often has excessive gross motor activity (e.g. excessive running-climbing, difficulty in sitting for long, restlessness).

Conduct Disorder

Disorders where the child's behavior is against social norms and values. The behaviors are repetitive and persistent. They violate rules. Their conduct is worse than ordinary mischief.

The common problems are:
1. Truancy (not attending school, spending time somewhere else).
2. Lying, stealing, substance abuse, breaking things, setting fire, often running away from home, gambling, poor peer group relations, fights with others, thefts outside home.
3. Does not accept responsibility and learn from past experiences and go on repeating the same mischief again and again. They often get caught by the police.

Sometimes this condition is also known as juvenile delinquency.

The cause of this disorder is mainly social, especially in the family. Parental rejection, harsh punishment, alcoholic or drug addict parents, illegitimate child, absent father are some of the causes.

School Refusal (School Phobia)

The reluctance or fear to go to school is seen among many children. This is known as school phobia or school refusal. School refusal may be associated with other neurotic symptoms such as shyness, fears and separation of anxiety (separation from mother). The mother may be over-protective and anxious.

The reasons for school phobia may be due to:
- Problems at school
- Problems at home
- Problems in the child.

Enuresis (Bedwetting)

The involuntary passage of urine in children over 5 years of age is termed as enuresis. Till five years of age, it may be regarded as physiological. Enuresis as a psychological problem more common among boys. The causes may be fear and anxiety in childhood, childhood depression, lack of toilet training, and being shy and inhibited.

Treatment includes proper bladder training. Antidepressant like imipramine 25 mg at night for 2–3 months is beneficial. Behavioral modification also may be helpful.

Child Abuse

Child Abuse is defined as physical or psychological damage to a child under the age of 18 that is sustained as a result of neglect or maltreatment.

The abuse may be physical, sexual and/or emotional. Physical abuse is also called battered child syndrome. Usually, the abuse is caused by a parent, a parent surrogate (e.g. step mother), a relative or an employer.

THE ROLE OF A NURSE IN CHILD MENTAL HEALTH PROBLEMS

It is the basic responsibility of a nurse to recognize a child with a mental health problem. It is done based on three features.

- The child's behavior is not appropriate for his age
- The child's behavior leads to disability
- The child's behavior is against social expectations.

The nurse, who happens to see a child with behavioral problems should understand that it is probably a reflection of the family's problems. Hence, understanding the family pathology is very essential.

The nurse, apart from carrying out the instructions from the doctor, can help children with mental health problems in the following ways:

- Finding out details of the underlying problem
- Trying to explain this to the concerned people and thereby reducing the problem
- Reassuring the parents
- Telling the parents not to give the child much attention when she is complaining
- Talk to the child in a sympathetic way and explain reasons to him
- Play therapy.

NURSING CARE FOR CHILD

- The child should achieve maximum possible living skills, self care skills, and adaptation to the environment
- Child maintains developmental progress

- Parents learn to adjust to the child's behavior and help in the developmental progress of the child
- Siblings and significant others will have reduced anxiety and realistic acceptance of the child
- Maintain progress in school
- Grow up into an adult with as much self care and living skills as possible.

MENTAL HEALTH PROBLEMS IN ADOLESCENTS

About 10–20% of adolescents in developed countries have educational, emotional, behavioral or social difficulties. The incidence is more in older adolescents living in deprived areas.

Adolescents' mental health problems can be classified into three groups.

1. Serious psychiatric disorders: Found in a few young people. These disorders include anxiety, depression, conduct disorders, alcoholism and drug abuse, psychosis like schizophrenia and eating disorders.
2. Disorders of mood and behavior: They are problematic but are not serious psychiatric disorders. They are quite common and influenced by social and family problems.
3. Transient reaction to adverse circumstances: Associated with more anxiety or sadness. Misbehavior, shyness, bedwetting, anxiety about friendship, school, sexual development and/or sexual preference and mixed feelings about independence and dependence. It may be etiological or symptomatic.

The incidence of depressive illness and attempted suicide rises dramatically during teenage years. In the later teens, attempted suicide is the commonest problem especially among girls.

SOCIAL FACTORS THAT AFFECT ADOLESCENTS

1. Poverty and overcrowding.
2. Parental attitude (e.g. inconsistency, extremes of discipline or neglect).
3. Parental illness or social problems, particularly maternal depression.
4. Marital disharmony in parents and family break-down
5. Poor schooling.
6. Repeated institutionalization (keeping him in hostels, boardings).

MANAGEMENT OF ADOLESCENT MENTAL HEALTH PROBLEMS

1. Individual treatment
   - Psychotherapy
   - Behavior therapy
   - Medication, e.g. antidepressants, if necessary.

2. Work with the family
   - Counseling and advice to family members
   - Family therapy
   - Marital therapy to parents.
3. Social and educational
   - A change of class or school
   - Career guidance
   - Job training schemes
   - Organized leisure activities
   - Encouragement to involve themselves in sports and games
   - Moral education.

In a developing country like India, the lifestyle of the population as a whole is undergoing a dramatic change. There is a tendency to mimic traditions of the West, at times blindly, with resulting frustrations. A widening gap between the conventional lifestyle and changing social values causes ongoing conflict, and the victim of this is the adolescent.

NURSING CARE FOR ADOLESNCENCE

- Youth suicide prevention education
- Life skills training
- Stable and supportive family
- Problem solving and emotional coping skills
- Teen building.

MENTAL HEALTH PROBLEMS IN WOMEN

Women are two to three times more at risk of developing mental disorders than men. One community survey in India reported the prevalence rate of mental illness among women to be 33.3 per 1000, while the corresponding figure for men was 15.7 per 1000.

Women are more prone to certain types of illness such as affective (mood) disorders, anxiety disorders, etc., thus, lending support to the view that the differences are qualitative rather than quantitative.

Why are Women More Prone to Develop Mental Disorders?

The feminine role: This may be due to social role of women. In a male dominated world, women are not getting the full opportunity to ventilate their feelings. Hence, they adopt a sick role which is more suitable for them to express themselves.

Genetics: Several disorders with a proven degree of heritability are commoner in females, e.g. affective disorder.

Endocrine factors: Women are prone to considerable degree of fluctuation in endocrine functions, and these have been important factors in the onset of mental illness.

Stressors: The stages of life cycle in women namely, puberty, menstruation, pregnancy, childbirth and menopause are all associated with endocrine changes and psychosocial stresses. During these stages, they are more vulnerable to psychiatric disturbances. The multiplicity of roles like daughter, wife and mother believed to predispose women to greater stress in our culture.

Age factor: Women at the late stage of their life (after 50 years) more prone to developing mental disorders due to multiple psychobiosocial factors. In adulthood, however, men and women suffer equally.

PSYCHIATRIC DISORDERS IN FEMALES

Affective (Mood) Disorders

They are commoner in women, especially so with depression. Roughly twice as many women as men are pathologically depressed.

Neurotic Disorders

These are reported to be higher among women. Anxiety and phobic disorders are twice as common in women as in men. Hysteria is believed to be almost exclusively confined to women.

Dementia

Women are at increased risk for the development of dementia, more because of their greater longevity.

Attempted Suicide

It is more common in females, especially in the age group of 15 to 30 years, whereas completed suicides are commoner in males. It is claimed that women are more prone to suicidal ideas and gestures during the phase of menstruation.

Anorexia Nervosa

This disorder is more common in adolescent girls.

Schizophrenia

Its prevalence is almost equal in both sexes, though some studies quote more males suffer than females. Alcoholism, drug abuse, personality disorders and criminality are much less common in females.

Specific Female Psychiatric Disorders

Premenstrual Syndrome

Behavior changes occurring in association with the menstrual cycle is well documented. The premenstrual syndrome, a cyclic recurrence of physical and psychological symptoms, may produce behavioral changes which are severe enough to disrupt interpersonal relationships and interfere with normal activities.

The psychological symptoms include anxiety, irritability and depression. The physical symptoms include breast tenderness, abdominal discomfort and a feeling of distension.

The etiology is uncertain. The biological basis of this disorder is claimed to be due to the fluctuation of hormonal and water levels.

This syndrome is widely treated with progesterone and also with oral contraceptives, bromocriptine, diuretics and psychotropic drugs like anti-depressants and anxiolytics.

Psychiatric Disorders that can occur after Childbirth (Postpartum or puerperal psychiatric disorders)

The increase of psychiatric disorders during the postpartum period is well known.

The possible causes are:

- A large drop in sex hormones in puerperium
- A rise in cortisol
- Changes in endorphin levels
- Chances of infections and complications during delivery
- Psychosocial conflict about playing the mother role or wife role
- Getting a child during an unwanted time or period, female child birth.

There is one in four chances of having a recurrence in the subsequent delivery.

The more common psychiatric problems in the postpartum period are:

- Maternity blues (mild depression)
- Puerperal depression of mild-to-moderate severity
- Puerperal (or) postpartum psychosis.

Maternity blues: In normal deliveries, between half and two-thirds experience brief episodes of irritability, lability of mood and episodes of crying. Symptoms reach the peak on third or fourth day after delivery. More common in primi. It is a short-lived condition.

Specific treatment is required and good, sympathetic nursing care will help these women. Supportive psychotherapy may be beneficial.

Puerperal depression: Less severe depressive disorders are much more common. Depression usually begins after the first two weeks of the puerperium. The total picture includes depression, tiredness, irritability and anxiety. Most patients recover after a few months. Antidepressants are effective in relieving the symptoms, psychological and social support will speed up recovery.

Puerperal psychosis: One in five hundred women after delivery may develop this disorder.

Three types of clinical picture are observed:
1. Acute organic psychosis
2. Affective psychosis
3. Schizophrenia-like psychosis.

Affective syndrome or a mixture of affective and schizophrenia-like psychosis are common.

Treatment is symptomatic, with antidepressants and/or antipsychotics. If necessary, ECT may be considered.

Nurses should see that the baby should remain with the mother to help maintain emotional attachment.

Menopause

In addition to the physical symptoms of flushing, sweating vaginal dryness, menopausal women often complain of headache, dizziness and multiple vague somatic complaints along with depression.

Depressive and anxiety-related symptoms at the time of menopause is sometimes known as involutional melancholia. Paranoid symptoms also occur in this condition.

The causes are:
1. Hormonal changes
    - Deficiency of estrogen.
2. Psychosocial
    - Changes in the woman's role during menopause
    - Children leaving home (Empty nest syndrome)
    - Relationship with her husband alters
    - Own parents become ill or die.

The treatment includes estrogen preparation and antidepressants and antianxiety drugs. Supportive and insight oriented psychotherapy will be beneficial.

MENTAL HEALTH PROBLEMS IN OLD AGE

Human ageing, a progressive loss of adaptability in an individual, is due to complex interplay between intrinsic (mainly genetic) and extrinsic (mainly environmental) factors. Longevity is not in all cases a blessing. Old age has always been fraught with problems that are intensified by the pressures of modern society and changing attitudes.

The definition of ageing depends upon how it is viewed from different perspectives. In India, it has been conventional to take 60th year as the point of turning old. The proportion of the people aged 60 or above constitutes 7% of the total population of India and number about 50 million today. This number is expected to each 60 million in 2000 AD.

MENTAL HEALTH PROBLEMS IN THE ELDERLY

Epidemiological studies have estimated the prevalence of mental morbidity among the aged at 89 per 1000, yielding a figure of nearly 4 millions in the country to be severely mentally ill.

Affective disorders (mostly) depression and to a lesser extent mania), paranoid states and organic mental disorders constitute the bulk of mental illness in the elderly. Depression is most frequent, with the prevalence rate of 60 per 1000. Dementias formed 20% of the total mental morbidity among the hospital aged patients.

Psychopathology increases with age. Organic mental disorders as well as functional psychoses increase in frequency with age. Suicide rates also rise sharply. Neurotic reactions are also a problem an old person's adaptability wanes to the extent that minor stresses precipitate depression and anxiety states. Depression, paranoid reactions and anxiety states should be as vigorously treated in the old as in the young.

Psychiatric illness in old age is not to be viewed in isolation. The mental health problems of the aged have to be examined with the prevailing social system. In view of the multiple system involvement, including psychiatric illness and also in view of the social, economic and the nutritional problems, the care of the elderly, to be meaningful, needs to be comprehensive.

The major mental health problems in old age are:

- Depression
- Dementia
- Delirium
- Paranoid disorder.

The three important factors associated with depression in old age are:

1. Emotional factors
   - Feeling lonely
   - Dissatisfaction with life
   - Self pity.
2. Physical factors
   - Deterioration in health
   - Difficulty in self care
   - Difficulty in mobility
   - Sensory deficits.
3. Socioeconomic factors
   - Widowed state
   - Loss of social status
   - Loss of income
   - Retirement
   - Bereavement.

DEPRESSION

Depression in old people may be present in ways which are rather different than those seen in younger people. The patient may be extremely agitated, with bizarre delusions concerning guilt, worthlessness or bodily disorder. Sometimes, the depression may be hidden behind an array of vague symptoms of anxiety or other neurotic complaints. When the symptoms are vague with no specific underlying cause the diagnosis could be depression. Hence, the use of the term masked depression is often used.

Sometimes the perplexity, the apparent lack of awareness and the total disregard of surroundings gives the picture of a dementing illness. This is called as pseudodementia.

Management of Depression in Elderly

Drugs play an important role in addition to psychological and social support in managing depression. Antidepressants with less anticholinergic and less cardiotoxic side-effects are preferred. Electroconvulsive therapy is safe, if given with proper care, in selected cases.

Steps to Minimize Depression in Elderly

1. Regular and periodic check-up of physical health.
2. Proper planning of retirement.
3. Low-cost health insurance schemes for old people.
4. Encouragement of traditional values and joint family system.
5. Advise to engage old people in religious activities and reading habits.

NURSING CARE FOR ELDERLY AGE

Role of nurse as
- Patient advocate
- Consultant
- Primary care provider.

Services for the elderly
- Primary care
- Hospital care
- Domiciliary services
- Residential care
- Day and outpatient care
- Psychogeriatric assessment unit.

Interventions
- Cognitive stimulation
- Promote a sense of calm and quiet
- Structure routine
- Focus on strengths and abilities
- Minimize disruptive behavior
- Minimal demands for complaint behavior
- Providing safety
- Relaxation therapy
- Supportive and counseling
- Health education to patient and family.

DEMENTIA

Dementia is identified as a major public health problem in old age. Dementia is an organic mental impairment with involvement of the brain. Dementia is defined as an acquired global impairment of the intellect, memory and personality without impairment of consciousness. Dementia is a dying mind in a living body. Dementia is not normal ageing or accelerated ageing, but a qualitative and quantitative change in intellectual function.

Causes of Dementia in Old Age (Primary cerebral cortical degenerations)

- Alzheimer's disease
- Pick's disease.

Cerebrovascular Disease

- Multi-infarct dementia

Primary Subcortical Degenerations

- Parkinson's disease
- Multiple system atrophy
- Huntington's disease
- Progressive supranuclear palsy
- 'Punch-drunk syndrome.

Cerebral Infection and Inflammation

- Neurosyphilis (GPI)
- Post-encephalitis
- Creutzfeldt-Jakob disease
- Multiple sclerosis.

Alcohol, Toxic and Metabolic

- Hypothyroidism
- Hypocalcemia
- Chronic hepatic encephalopathy
- Chronic uremia and dialysis
- Vitamin B12 deficiency
- Pellagra
- Malabsorption syndrome.

Tumors and Hydrocephalous

- Meningiomas
- Benign gliomas
- Parapituitary tumors
- Intraventricular tumors
- Pineal and midbrain tumors
- Secondary deposits
- Subdural hematomas
- Giant aneurysms
- Aqueduct stenosis
- Communicating hydrocephalous.

After excluding secondary dementia the most common the primary dementias are:

1. Alzheimer's disease and
2. Multi-infarct dementia.

The Diagnostic Features of Dementia

1. Demonstrable evidence of impairment in short- and long-term memory.
2. Impairment in abstract thinking, judgment, higher cortical functions and personality change.
3. Disturbances that significantly interfere with work and social activities.
4. Not a part of delirium that is, there is no change in consciousness.
5. Evidence of organic change.

Management of Dementia in Elderly

Drugs have a limited role to play in the management of dementia. Drugs are helpful in managing associated psychosis, behavioral problem and to improve the cerebral blood circulation.

Psychosocial Management of Demented Elderly

Dementia is often accompanied by a behavior supervened by psychotic symptoms. Management in addition to psychopharmacology should include a totally psychosocial approach.

Psychosocial intervention in dementia includes:

- Behavioral methods
- Milieu therapy
- Activity engagement
- Physical exercise
- Problem-oriented approach
- Reality orientation
- Organization of psychiatric services.

Behavioral methods: Much rehabilitation is based on the analysis of problems and the setting of goals. Behavioral methods share these principles, but add specific procedures to modify particular aspects of behavior. Lately, these methods have been directed to improve deficits of memory, e.g. use of lists and reminders and by practice.

Methods have been identified for training patients with problem in eating, continence or social skills. Reality orientation therapy, which is intended to reduce confusion and improve behavior.

As the illness progresses the patient may be incapable of managing activities of daily living. Activities which entail potential danger must be avoided, such as driving, using power tools, smoking and using a stove. Leaving the house unaccompanied may also be a potential risk. The patient's daily routine should be continuously monitored, simplified and regularized to maintain well-learned behaviors and to minimize stressful changes.

The family and other caregivers should be fully involved in these changes. Dementia affects the entire family. Education of the patients and the family is essential.

Supportive psychotherapy to demented patients, with clearly defined aims may be required.

Organization of supportive services for demented patients, wherever available would go a long way in sharing the burden.

DELIRIUM

Delirium is again a common psychological disturbance in the Elderly. It is an organic brain syndrome characterized by impairment in consciousness, orientation, attention and behavior; onset is acute fluctuating in course. Elderly are particularly vulnerable to the development of delirium in association with any physical illness. Often it occurs in the general medical ward.

Etiological organic factors could be identified in 80–95% of reported cases of delirium in the elderly.

The commonest causes of delirium in elderly are:

- Drugs
- Metabolic causes
- Malnutrition
- Respiratory diseases
- Cardiovascular diseases
- Liver diseases
- Cerebrovascular disorders 8, fever
- Alcohol
- Trauma
- Fever.

Management of Delirium

In the elderly management of delirium includes assessment of basic causes, treating the causes, maintaining fluid and electrolyte balance and good nursing care. Minimal doses of antipsychotic drugs for a short time can be given.

Nursing Care of Delirium

Keep the patient in a comfortable, quiet, well lighted place. Less stimuli is advisable. Reassure the patient and be supportive, orient the patient to time, place and people frequently. Have a consistent sympathetic and understanding nursing care.

PARANOID DISORDERS

Apart from dementia, paranoid disorders (delusional disorders) occur occasionally in old age. Paranoid disorder occurring in old age is at times known as paraphrenia, more common among elderly women.

Clinical Features Include

Suspiciousness, persecutory delusion, agitation, restlessness, depression and insomnia.

Treatment with mild dose of major tranquilizers is beneficial.

NURSING CARE OF ELDERLY WITH MENTAL HEALTH PROBLEM

The nurse should understand that most old people are dependents and have a feeling of insecurity. The nurse should also understand the common symptoms of senility like:

1. Change in attention span.
2. Memory loss for recent events and names.
3. Altered intellectual capacity.
4. Diminished ability to respond to others.

The long-term nursing goal is to help the patient in reducing hopelessness and helplessness. Short-term goals are to educate the patient to preserve their self image and preserve their abilities to perform. The nurse should reassure and encourage the patient to reduce depression and feelings of isolation and educate them to correct sensory deficit (e.g. cataract operation of eye will improve their vision and reduce their dependency). Teach them to take care of physical illnesses, which are common in elderly. If possible encourage them to do simple physical exercises like walking which will enhance blood flow.

Chapter

22

Common Psychophysiological Disorders (Psychosomatic Disorders)

Psychophysiological disorders are a group of disorders in which emotional factors have a demonstrable role in the etiology. Severe stress may play an etiological role in the development of certain physical diseases. They are also known as stress related disorders.

The word psychosomatic means mind and body just as the emotion of anxiety can produce sweating, palpitation and tremor, severe emotions of long duration can produce permanent damage in the body system. Most of these disorders are treated in a general hospital set up rather than in psychiatric hospital.

Possible progression of psychosomatic disorders
Prolonged anxiety leads to persistent psychophysiological reactions, which causes structural alteration, cellular diseases, and functional impairment which may lead to psychosomatic disorders.

PSYCHOSOCIAL THEORIES

1. Individuals exhibit specific physiological responses to certain emotions, e.g. in response to the emotion of anger, one person may experience peripheral vasoconstriction, resulting in an increase in blood pressure. The same emotion in another individual my evoke the response of cerebral vasodilation, manifesting a migraine headache.
2. Personality Theory: Individuals with specific personality traits are predisposed to certain disease processes. Personality traits may form a possible relationship but cannot be the total cause for the disease.

   Personality characteristic psychosomatic disorder dependence:
   - Asthma
   - Repressed anger
   - Peptic ulcer and hypertension
   - Aggressive, ambitious type of personality
   - Coronary heart disease

  - Compulsive and perfectionist
  - Migraine
  - Self-sacrificing and inhibited
  - Rheumatoid arthritis and ulcerative colitis.
3. Learning Theory: Conditioned responses reinforced by secondary gains.
4. Family Dynamic Theory: Pathogenic family patterns in childhood predispose psychosomatic disorders. Stressful and conflicting interpersonal relationships among family members also may be a cause.
5. Biological theory: Psychosomatic disorders occur when the body is exposed to prolonged stress, producing a number of physiological effects under direct control of the pituitary adrenal axis.

Genetic predisposition also influences which organ system will be affected and determines the psychosomatic disorder.

COMMON PSYCHOSOMATIC DISORDERS

- Cardiovascular system, coronary heart disease
- Essential hypertension
- Respiratory system, bronchial asthma
- Hyperventilation syndrome
- Gastrointestinal system, peptic ulcer
- Ulcerative colitis
- Irritable bowel syndrome
- Musculoskeletal rheumatoid arthritis
- Headaches vascular—migraine headache
- Muscle contraction– tension headache
- Skin eczema
- Endocrine hyperthyroidism
- Diabetes mellitus
- Premenstrual syndrome, menopausal disorder
- Eating disorders, anorexia nervosa
- Bulimia
- Obesity
- Psychogenic pain.

SOME IMPORTANT PSYCHOSOMATIC DISORDERS

Asthma

The possibility that a psychosomatic component may have a role to play in asthma has been observed for a long time. It is observed that asthmatics manifest more negative emotions than normal people. Hostility, anxiety, depression, a sense of helplessness, personality disorders and a decreased competence were common features in asthmatics. Increased attacks of asthma were reported in the morning during crying, shouting or laughing.

In the management of asthma, along with medications, supportive psychotherapy, relaxation exercise and yoga could play a vital role in the long-term control of the disease.

Coronary Heart Disease

A link has been claimed between coronary heart disease and type A behavior pattern. The behavior pattern of type A personality includes excessive ambition, high performance standards, persistent urgency, competitiveness, aggressiveness and hostility. Hence, type A personality persons have a high risk for developing coronary heart disease. The treatment includes, apart from medication, insight-oriented psychotherapy and teaching and teaching a better way of relaxation in between their work.

It is also reported in various studies that persons suffering from myocardial infarction are exposed to stressful events prior to the onset of their attacks.

Peptic Ulcer (Acid Peptic Disease)

Clinical observation and experimental evidence have indicated that stress produces increased adrenocortical secretion which results in the the initiation, formation and severity of gastric ulcers.

Irritable Bowel Syndrome (IBS)

The symptoms of IBS include abdominal pain, a sensation of distension, altered bowel habits, passage of mucus and a sense of incomplete evacuation after defecation. Persons suffering from IBS are reported to be having more psychological symptoms and illness.

The psychological symptoms associated with IBS are anxiety, depression, obsessional characteristics, multiple somatic symptoms and "illness behavior". The psychiatric illnesses associated with IBS are depressive disorder, generalized anxiety disorder, panic disorder and phobic disorder.

MANAGEMENT

Management includes symptomatic treatment of the disease, supportive psychotherapy and teaching measures to cope with stress and stress reducing measures like relaxation therapy.

NURSING CARE IN PSYCHOSOMATIC DISORDERS

The nurse should establish a good therapeutic relationship with the patient. She should first understand the exact problem, the basic personality type, the family background, the stress inducing situations, the positive and negative qualities of the individual, etc. This will provide a base for better assessment and management.

The nurse should help the patient to learn to cope with his stresses more effectively. Encourage patient to discuss his problems. The patient may need assistance with problem solving, verbalization of feelings in a non-threatening environment. This may help the patient to come to terms with unresolved issues. Patient may be unaware of the relationship between physical symptoms and emotional problems. This should be clarified.

- Therapy is facilitated by considering areas of strength and utilizing them to the patient benefit
- Positive reinforcement enhances self-esteem and encourages' repetition of desirable behavior
- The feeling of acceptance by others increases self-esteem, hence the nurse should accept the patient as he is
- Encourage family participation in the therapy. Family may require assistance in this process
- Patients are encouraged to come out of the sick role
- Teach the patient assertiveness technique. The nurse should teach the patient adaptive methods of stress management such as relaxation techniques, physical exercises, meditation, breathing exercise and yoga. Use of these adaptive techniques may decrease the appearance of physical symptoms in response to stress.

ROLE OF NURSES

- Assess the body change with which the client is preoccupied. If the client's normal appearance or functioning has changed, help the client to explore his feelings about the change
- Collaborate with the client to identify misperceptions regarding body image
- Provide accurate feedback in a direct, nonthreatening manner
- Encourage the client to participate in body-image group activities and movement therapy activities
- Encourage and reinforce the client's independent, self-care activities, participating or assisting only when necessary
- Encourage the client to use cognitive restructuring strategies
- Acknowledge the client's pain perception as a real event

- Collaborate with the multidisciplinary treatment team to develop a comprehensive consistent approach to the client's somatic complaints
- Teach the client assertiveness skills and incorporate these skills in role-playing sessions
- Consult with occupational, physical, recreational, and movement therapist to establish appropriate treatment plans and to determine adaptive coping strategies
- Help the client to regain the ability to perform normal daily functions
- Provide the client with opportunities for increased socialization.

Chapter

23

Community Psychiatry

Community psychiatry is the branch of psychiatry that develops and maintains organized programs for the promotion of mental health, the prevention and treatment of mental disorders and the habilitation of the psychiatric patient.

CONCEPT OF COMMUNITY CARE

Community care involves a community health service which provides comprehensive care and treatment for a defined population.

The two essential aspects are:
1. There should be continuity of care.
2. The available services are to be integrated.

The basic requirement of community care involves.
1. Treatment close to the patient's home.
2. Comprehensive services.
3. Multi-disciplinary team approach.
4. Continuity of care.
5. Consumer participation.
6. Program evaluation and research.

The two main components of community psychiatry are:
1. Promotion of positive mental health.
2. Prevention of mental illness.

MENTAL HEALTH

Health is not merely absence of disease. It is a condition of physical, mental and social wellbeing.

One should strive to attain the highest possible level of health that will permit one to lead a socially and economically productive life. Mental health does not mean mere absence of mental illness. There should be some positive qualities in every human being to contribute to his or her society. The individual must have a sense of wellbeing.

Mental health and physical health are interrelated and interdependent. A sound mind resides in a sound body.

DEFINITION OF MENTAL HEALTH

WHO defines mental health as "The capacity of an individual to form harmonious relationship, with others and to actively participate in the changes in the social environment."

Meininger defines mental health as, "The adjustment of a human being to the world and to each other, with a maximum of effectiveness and happiness."

Mental health is an ability to maintain:

1. An even temper.
2. An alert intelligence.
3. A socially considerate behavior.
4. A happy disposition.

Good adjustment is the basis for positive mental health. Mental health is an individual matter. It involves an individual human mind. A social environment or culture may be conducive either to sickness or health, but the quality produced is characteristic only of a person. Mental health is a state in which one's potential capacities are fully realized. Maturity, as adjustment can also be regarded as mental health.

The terms mature, well adjusted, and psychologically healthy are often used as synonyms. There should be a positive approach towards attaining mental health.

CHARACTERISTICS OF A MENTALLY HEALTHY PERSON

1. A mentally healthy person is free from internal conflicts. He is not at war with himself.
2. He is well adjusted; i.e. he is able to get along well with others. He is able to form effective relationships. He accepts criticism and is not easily upset.
3. He searches for an entity.
4. He has a strong sense of self-esteem.
5. He knows himself his needs, problems and goals. This is known as self-actualization.
6. He has good control over his behavior.
7. He is productive.
8. He faces problems and tries to solve them intelligently. He is able to cope with stress and anxiety. Mental health is the full and harmonious functioning of the whole personality.

THE REQUIREMENTS OF MENTAL HEALTH

a. Full expression of potential, personality, etc.
b. Harmonization.
c. The direction to a common end of native and acquired potentials.

Living in a stress-free environment will pave the way for mentally healthier and happier life. In general, mental health can be achieved through many ways including individual treatment, treatment of families, educational programs, etc. Sound behavioral patterns can be encouraged and reinforced in a well established social network. Widespread mental health is the need of the hour. Mental health is a positive science in that it aims at a condition of healthy mindedness.

PREVENTION OF MENTAL ILLNESS

The prevention of mental illness is based on public health principles and has been divided into:

1. Primary prevention.
2. Secondary prevention.
3. Tertiary prevention.

The aim of prevention is to decrease, the onset (incidence), duration (prevalence) and residual disability of mental disorder.

Primary Prevention

Primary prevention involves the promotion of general mental health and protection against the occurrence of specific diseases. Primary prevention aims to prevent the onset of a disease or disorder, thereby reducing the incidence (number of new cases occurring in a specific period of time).

Measures for primary prevention include:

1. Elimination of etiological agents.
2. Reducing risk factors.
3. Enhancing host resistance or interfering with disease transmission.
4. Reducing stress factors.
5. Counseling
    - Student's counseling
    - Marriage counseling
    - Sex counseling
    - Genetic counseling.
6. Special centers
    - Child guidance center
    - Crisis intervention center
    - Geriatric center
7. Mental health education.

Mental health promotion programs should not be considered scientifically based, medical matters, but rather with the notion of recreation, entertainment and moral upliftment.

Mental Health Education

Among health problems, mental illnesses are poorly understood by the general public. The message of prevention, early recognition and effective treatment should reach them· Repeated efforts to give correct information will lead to a positive change and the misconceptions about mental illnesses removed.

Secondary Prevention

Early identification and effective treatment of an illness or disorder, with the goal of reducing the prevalence (total number of existing cases in a year) is the aim of secondary prevention.

The essential components of secondary prevention are:

1. Population screening.
2. Crisis intervention services.
3. Mental health education.

The paramedical professionals have to be trained to understand mental illnesses, identify them early, treat many of them and the rest to a specialist. Mental health education aims at educating the public to recognize mental illness at an early stage and seek help.

Secondary prevention of mental illness is generally accepted as an important aspect of mental health services.

Tertiary Prevention or Rehabilitation

This aims to reduce the prevalence of residual defect or disability due to illness or disorder. Tertiary prevention involves rehabilitation after defect and disability have been fixed. Human behavior can be changed, by gradual shaping, into completely new responses. This can be achieved by behavior therapy methods like token economy. Modem tertiary prevention of mental illness or rehabilitation of the seriously disabled mentally ill persons is one of the great success stories of psychiatry.

Community mental health addresses on how to promote mental health and prevent various forms of mental disorders and a variety of interventions.

- Promotion
- Preventive, curative, and right
- Rehabilitative: According to mental health experts in the field community mental health will provide mental health care in the community as opposed to institutional settings

- Focus services on a total community or population rather than on an individual patients
- Focus on preventive and promotive services as distinguished from therapeutic ones
- Provide continuity and comprehensiveness of services rather than the care based on illness episodes
- Provide indirect services such as consultation and mental health education rather than direct service to patients
- Plan community involvement to establish priorities for needed mental health services
- Develop and train new mental health workers who could provide basic mental health care.

The nurses role which perform in the community mental health set up are:

Consultant role: Advisor to other professionals about type and level of nursing required to a client group.

Clinician role: Delivering the nursing care to clients in the community.

Therapeutic role: Psychotherapy and behavior therapy.

- Educator: Mental health education
- Assessor and researcher role: Assess the outcome of ongoing care programs
- Trainers: Training of paraprofessionals, community leaders, and school teachers, etc.
- Manager/administrator: Management of resources and work priorities, planning and coordination of the development of future patterns of community care
- Domiciliary care: Home visit services like administration of medication, assessment, monitoring side effects of drugs and counseling to the client and family members
- Liaison role: Nurses working in the community helps the client and family members by bridging the gap between the client and the hospital, client and the employers, etc.
- Prevention role: Nurses can play a vital role in prevention of mental disorder at three levels;
- Primary prevention
- Secondary prevention
- Tertiary prevention.

Chapter

24

Treatment of Mental Disorders

Patients suffering from physical illnesses are given specific treatment because the causes are specific and the signs and syndromes are specific. The doctor generally knows how the treatment works, and the patient co-operates with the doctors, and nurses order to get better. In psychiatric hospital, the treatment may not be so specific and most patients are given more than one treatment. These treatment methods vary from patient to patient. Some psychiatric patients do not want treatment and may not co-operate with the doctors and nurses. Some do not realize that they are ill and may actively resist all forms of treatment.

The nurse has an extremely important role to play in the treatment of the mentally ill. She has always much closer contact with the patient than any other members of the hospital team. She also has a greater opportunity to get to know him and report on his improvement. Her actions, attitudes, and skills to help him to deal with his problems are themselves an essential part of his treatment.

The treatment for psychiatric disorders can be divided into two types-physical methods of treatment and psychological methods of treatment. Most patients will be treated with one or more methods of treatment.

Physical methods of treatment include:

1. Drug treatment, (Pharmacotherapy)
2. Somatic therapies include:
   A. Electroconvulsive therapy (ECT)
   B. Stimulation techniques.

DRUG TREATMENT PHARMACOTHERAPY

Drugs used in the management of psychiatric disorders are together known as psychotropic drugs. The following is the classification of various drugs in psychiatry:

- Antipsychotic drugs
- Antidepressants
- Mood stabilizers

- Antianxiety drugs
- Anticholinergics drugs
- Psychostimulants
- Cognitive enhancers
- Others.

PRINCIPLES OF MANAGEMENT

Principles of Pharmacological Management

- Initiate after careful assessment of diagnosis and medical condition
- Careful choice of the drug
- Monitor for side effects and possible toxicity
- Review for effectiveness
- Change, only if required
- Plan duration of regime
- Consider discontinuation
- Avoid unduly long prescription.

I. Common prescription errors
   - Irrational polypharmacy
   - Sub-therapeutic doses
   - Pre-formulated combinations
   - Medication continued without review of the need
   - Tranquilizers for all situations.

II. Myths about psychotropic drugs
   - All are "Sleeping pills"
   - All are "Tranquilizers" only
   - All are "Addictive"
   - Have to be taken for lifetime/indefinitely.

ANTIPSYCHOTIC DRUGS

Drugs used in the management of various psychotic disorders (severe mental illnesses) are known as antipsychotic drugs. Earlier they were also known as major tranquillizers or neuroleptics. The era of antipsychotic pharmacotherapy began with the discovery of chlorpromazine by Delay and Deniker in 1952. Since then a number of antipsychotic drugs have developed with differences in their mechanism of actions effects and side effects profile.

Indications for the use of antipsychotics:

1. Schizophrenia.
2. Acute psychotic disorders.

3. Organic mental disorders (in low dose).
4. Postpartum psychosis.
5. Bipolar disorder—in mania and as a mood stabilizer.
6. Low dose in anorexia nervosa, in attention deficit hyperactive disorder, behavioral problem in mental retardation and in depression with psychotic features.

The following are the two important groups of antipsychotics:

1. First Generation Antipsychotics (Conventional or typical antipsychotics)—FGA

   These drugs mainly act as an antipsychotic by blocking D_2 receptors. They also block muscarinic, anticholinergic, histaminic and alpha 1 receptors. All these conventional or typical antipsychotics are capable of producing Extrapyramidal syndromes (EPS) and often Tardive dyskinesia (TD) from D_2 receptors blocking property especially in nigrostriatal pathway.

   Conventional antipsychotic agents and their dosage range.

Generic name	Dosage range (mg/day)
1. Chlorpromazine	50–1200
2. Thioridazine	150–800
3. Trifluoperazine	5–30
4. Haloperidol	2–60
5. Pimozide	4–8

Side effects of FGA (conventional or typical antipsychotic)

1. Anticholinergic effects—Dry mouth, blurred vision, constipation and urinary retention.
2. Sedation.
3. Orthostatic hypotension.
4. Photosensitivity (Skin rashes).
5. Endocrine effects—Amenorrhea and milky secretion from the breast (in women).
   Due to increased prolactin level.
   Weight gain.
   Decreased libido, gynecomastia.
6. Reduction of seizure threshold (occurrence of fits).
7. Extrapyramidal side-effects (EPS)
   a. Pseudoparkinsonism (tremor, shuffling gait, rigidity, drooling of saliva, mask like face)—may appear in 1–5 days following antipsychotic medications.
   b. Acute dystonia—occurs soon after the initiation of treatment. Dystonia is the sustained muscle contraction and the manifestations

include torticollis, tongue protrusion, grimacing, opisthotonus and oculogyric crisis. Treatment includes administration of parenteral anticholinergic agents like promethazine (phenergan).

c. Akathisia is a subjective feeling of restlessness leading to inability to sit still. The person cannot sit or stand in a particular position for sometime, is restless and sense of wanting to jump. Its starts appearing in the first 2 weeks of treatment. Injection promethazine or injection lorazepan may be beneficial.

d. Tardive dyskinesia (TD) is a long-term complication of antipsychotics mainly with D_2 antagonists and is hypothesized to be due to supersensitization of D_2 receptors in nigrostriatal pathway resulting from prolonged D_2 blockage. The most common dyskinesias include chewing and sucking (Oro-bucco-linguo-masticatory) movements, grimacing and choreoathetoid movements. Till date, no effective treatment of TD is available.

e. Neuroleptic malignant syndrome (NMS) is a rare but extremely serious complication of antipsychotics especially with high potency D_2 antagonists like haloperidol. Symptoms include fluctuating consciousness, hyperthermia, muscle rigidity and automatic instability. Laboratory findings include increased white blood cell count, CPK and serum creatinine. Treatment is mainly supportive. The offending drug should be discontinued. Electrolytes and fluid balance should be maintained. Dantrolene, bromocriptine and amantadine have been tried. Mortality rate is quite high (20–40%).

SECOND GENERATION ANTIPSYCHOTICS—SGA (NOVEL OR ATYPICAL ANTIPSYCHOTICS)

Since, the first generation or conventional antipsychotics have limited efficacy and lot of side effects, the SGA have come into the active management of psychotic disorders in the reason past.

The Advantages of SGA (Atypicals)

- Beneficial effects on both positive and negative symptoms
- Low incidence of EPS, TD and NMS
- Low stimulation of prolactin secretion
- Effective in treatment resistant cases
- Dopamine blocking actions is mainly on Mesolimbic pathway, avoiding Nigrostriatal pathway
- Atypicals have low affinity towards D_2 receptors but also to D_1 and other receptors like serotonin ($5HT_2$)
- The atypicals act on SDA concepts—both serotonin and dopamine antagonist actions.

Atypical antipsychotic	Initial dose (mg)	Standard dose (mg/ day)	Dosing frequency	Max dose	Advantages
Clozapine	25–50	300–600	BID	900	Effective in refractory schizophrenia. Lowestrisk of extra-pyramidal symptoms (EPS)
Olanzapine	5–10	15–20	QD to BID	20	Well tolerated Approved for acute mania
Quetiapine	25–50	400–600	BID	800	Well tolerated lowest EPS risk
Risperidone	1–2	4–8	QD to BID	16	Well tolerated. Well defined dose range
Atypical antipsychotic	Initial dose (mg)	Standard dose (mg/ day)	Dosing frequency	Max dose	Advantages
Ziprasidone	40–80	80–160	BID	160	No weight gain Injectable form
Aripiprazole	10–15	15	QD	30	Dopamine system stabilizer
Amisulpride	100–200	300–800	BID	800	Minimum EPS no weight gain
Zotepine	50–150	100–300		300	

COMPARISON OF NEWER (SECOND GENERATION) ATYPICAL ANTIPSYCHOTICS

Side effects profile of SGA (Atypicals)

- Compared to conventional antipsychotic they have very low incidence of EPS, TD and NMS

- Weight gain - common especially in olanzapine, clozapine and zotepine
- Blood dyscrasias—Agranulocytosis a rare side effects with clozapine–periodic WBC and absolute neutrophil count to be done
- Diabetes—Atypicals especially drugs like olanzapine, clozapine and risperidone may increase blood sugar. Often they accelerate the already existing diabetes mellitus or occasionally induce new diabetic cases
- Metabolic syndrome—Glucose dysregulation (Diabetes), hypertension, dyslipidemia (increased triglyceride) and obesity constitute the metabolic syndrome. Atypicals like clozapine, olanzapine, risperidone and zotepine may induce metabolic syndrome
- Epilepsy in few cases. Atypicals like clozapine and zotepine may induce seizure.

DEPOT ANTIPSYCHOTICS (LONG-ACTING ANTIPSYCHOTICS)

Depot preparations are often preferable in:

1. Maintenance treatment of long-term psychotic disorders.
2. Treatment resistant cases
3. Unwilling and non-cooperative patients.
4. Patients with poor drug compliance.

The following are some of the depot preparations:

Generic name	Dosage range (mg)
Injection Fluphenazine deconate	25 mg once in 2 weeks
Injection Haloperidol deconate	50 mg once in 2–4 weeks
Injection Risperidone—long-acting	25 mg once in 2–4 weeks
Injection Flupenthixol	40 mg once in 1–4 weeks
Injection Zuclopenpixol	200 mg once in 1–4 weeks

ANTIDEPRESSANTS

The drugs use in the treatment of depression and related disorders are known as antidepressants.

The following are the group of antidepressants:

A. Tricyclic antidepressants (TCA).
B. Selective serotonin reuptake inhibitors (SSRI).
C. Monoamine oxidase inhibitors (MAOI).
D. Others.

INDICATIONS FOR ANTIDEPRESSANTS

1. Depressive disorders—Severe depression, moderate depression, dysthymia (mild depression), atypical depression, bipolar depression,

postpartum depression, adjustment disorder with depression, depression in organic mental disorders, depression in psychosis.
2. Neurotic and stress related disorders—Panic disorders, obsessive compulsive disorder (OCD), phobic disorders, post-traumatic stress disorder (PTSD), somatoform disorders, acute stress reaction.
3. Eating disorders—Bulimia.
4. Sleep disorders—Insomnia and parasomnias.
5. Pain disorders—Fibromyalgia, neuropathic pain disorders.
6. In children—ADHD, school refusal, nocturnal enuresis, childhood depression.

TRICYCLIC ANTIDEPRESSANTS (TCA)

Depression is considered to be due to a low level of neurotransmitters like, serotonin and noradrenaline at the synapse. These drugs block the reuptake of both 5HT and NA, there by increasing the availability of these amines.

COMMONLY USED TRICYCLIC ANTIDEPRESSANTS

Generic name	Daily dosage range (mg)
1. Imipramine	50-300
2. Amitriptyline	50-300
3. Nortriptyline	50-150
4. Doxepin	50-300
5. Dothepin	50-300
6. Trimipramine	50-200
7. Clomipramine	50-200

Side Effects

1. Anti-cholinergic effects—dry mouth, blurred vision, constipation, urinary retention.
2. Sedation
3. Orthostatic hypotension
4. Cardiac—Tachycardia, arrhythmias
5. May induce paralytic ileus and convulsions: Precipitate glaucoma.
6. High risk for overdose and poisoning.

SELECTIVE SEROTONIN REUPTAKE INHIBITORS (SSRIs)

Advantages of SSRIs

- The most preferred antidepressant in the present day management of depression

- Widely used in all the depressive disorders and related disorders and they are safely used in children and elderly and with associated psychical disorders—because of their safety, better efficacy and low side effects profile
- Simple dose regime—hence primary care physician and specialist can widely use
- Early onset of antidepressant actions
- The danger of over dose and poisoning is almost nil.

MECHANISM OF ACTION

Unlike TCA, SSRI have selective serotonin reuptake inhibition without interfering with NA.

Commonly used SSRI's

Generic name	Daily dosage range (mg)
1. Fluoxetine	20–80
2. Citalopram	10–40
3. Escitalopram	10–20
4. Sertraline	50–100
5. Paroxetine	12.5–50
6. Fluvoxamine	50–200

Side effects of SSRI's

- Yawning, nausea, vomiting
- Agitation and restlessness
- Sexual dysfunction—especially ejaculatory dysfunction
- Rarely sedation, Parkinson like features, convulsion
- In extremely high dose may produce Serotonin syndrome (Toxicity, confusion, high fever, myoclonic jerks, etc.)
- SSRI discontinuation syndrome—develop rarely after 3–5 days of stopping SSRI—electric shock like sensations, dizziness, insomnia, GI tract symptoms, etc.

OTHER NEW ANTIDEPRESSANT DRUGS

A. Serotonin and noradrenaline reuptake inhibitors (SNRI's)
   1. Venlafaxine (75–300 mg/day).
   2. Desvenlafaxine (50–100 mg/day).
   3. Duloxetine (20–60 mg/day).
   4. Milnacipran (50–100 mg/day).

5. Bupropion (75-450 mg/day).
6. Trazodone (50-150 mg/day).

All the above drugs are dual actions reuptake inhibitors. That is they are selectively inhibiting both 5HT and NA. Hence, they are more efficient as an antidepressant. Duloxetine inhibit all the three amines namely, 5HT, NA and also DA. The duloxetine and milnacipran are also useful in the pain disorders like fibromyalgia and neuropathic pain disorders.

B. Alpha 2 adrenoceptor antagonists
   Mirtazapine—an antidepressant involving 5HT, NA and also anti-histaminergic and $\alpha 2$ antagonists.
   Relatively sedative dose 15-30 mg/day.

Monoamine oxidase inhibitors (MAOI's)
These molecules act by inhibiting MAO enzymes A and B. They are not commonly used because of its toxic, at time serious side effects like cheese reactions. Rarely indicated in other drugs resistant depressive cases.

MAOI molecules are not available in India.

MOOD STABILIZERS

Mood stabilizers are drugs used in bipolar disorder to stabilize the fluctuating extreme mood states. Mood stabilizers are useful to

1. Prevent or to minimize future episodes of mania or depression or to some extent.
2. Reduce the severity of these mood disorders.

The following are the important mood stabilizers:

1. Lithium.
2. Anticonvulsants
   a. Valproate
   b. Carbamazepine
   c. Oxcarbazepine
   d. Lamotrigine
   e. Topiramate.

Lithium

Lithium Carbonate:

Lithium is the first mood stabilizer to be used in psychiatry. Lithium is effective in treating cases of mania. It is a potential anti-manic agent apart from being a mood stabilizer.

Lithium is thought to enhance the reuptake of the biogenic amines in the brain, thus, lowering their levels in the body. Another theory suggest that it alters sodium metabolism within nerve and vessel cells.

Indications of Lithium

1. Prevention and treatment of mania, hypomania, and bipolar disorders.
2. In the treatment of recurrent depression.
3. Severe depressive patients with suicidal tendency.

Dosage of lithium is 900–1200 mg/day in divided doses.

The effective therapeutic level is 0.8 to 1.2 millimol/L.

If the serum lithium goes below the therapeutic level the action will not be significant. If it goes above the therapeutic level it may produce adverse effects and if serum lithium level goes beyond 2.0 millimol/L that may produce toxic effects and is a dangerous emergency condition. Hence, whenever a patient is on lithium, it is always necessary to have frequent monitoring of serum lithium level.

Side effects of lithium: Nephrogenic diabetes insipidus, interstitial nephritis, reversible hypothyroidism.

Lithium toxicity: Can occur when serum lithium level goes beyond 2 millimol/L. Inadequate fluid intake, diarrhea, dehydration, increased sweating in summer may cause this toxicity. The toxic effects include tremor, ataxia, dysarthria, nystagmus, renal impairment, and convulsion.

Management: Periodic monitoring of serum lithium level, monitoring BUN and serum creatinine, stop lithium when symptoms of toxicity occur, increase the sodium and fluid intake, dialysis, if necessary.

Anticonvulsants

Almost all the anticonvulsants act as mood stabilizers.

A. Sodium valproate is the most widely used anticonvulsants for the effective management of bipolar disorder.
   Dosage: 500 to 2000 mg/day.
   Weight gain, hair loss, polycystic ovary disease are the common adverse effects.
B. Carbamazepine is an effective anticonvulsant and is also found to be an effective mood stabilizer.
   Dosage: 400–1200 mg/day.
   Adverse Effects: Gastrointestinal tract disturbances, double vision, nystagmus, ataxia. Apart from this, life-threatening aplastic anemia, and agranulocytosis may occur. This should be immediately taken care off.
C. Oxcarbazepine is an anticonvulsant, also useful as an antimanic agent under mood stabilizer. It is slightly an improved form of carbamazepine. Some of the side effects of carbamazepine may not occur with oxcarbazepine.
   Dosage: 400–1200 mg/day.

D. Lamotrigine: Lamotrigine is an anticonvulsant may also be used as a mood stabilizer. Lamotrigine is much useful in bipolar disorder where depressive episodes are more frequent than manic episodes.
Dosage: 100–200 mg/day.

E. Topiramate: A novel anticonvulsant. It is also useful as a mood stabilizer.
Dosage: 200–400 mg/day.
All the mood stabilizers may also useful in the manic episode of bipolar disorder. It is very essential to recognize very early the symptoms of mania or depression and accordingly treat them with mood stabilizers. Thus, all mood stabilizers act as antimanic agents.

ANXIOLYTICS AND HYPNOTICS

Anxiolytics: They are also known as antianxiety drugs or minor tranquilizers. They are effective in reducing the anxiety in anxiety disorders and also facilitate sleep. Majority of the anxiolytics come under the group of benzodiazepines. They act by enhancing GABA function in the neurons.

Classification of Anxiolytics and Hypnotics

	Dosage
I. Benzodiazepines	
• Chlordiazepoxide	20–100 mg/day
• Diazepam	5–20 mg/day
• Oxazepam	30–120 mg/day
• Alprazolam	0.5–4 mg/day
• Nitrazepam	5–20 mg/day
• Clonazepam	1–4 mg/day
• Midazolam	5–50 mg/day
• Flurazepam	5–30 mg at night (Only parenteral)
II. Non-benzodiazepines	
1. Buspirone	20–30 mg/day
2. Beta-blockers	10–40 mg/day
III. Hypnotics:	
• Zolpidem	5–10 mg at night
• Zopiclone	1–2 mg at night

Benzodiazepines
Inhibit GABA. They act mainly on the reticular and limbic system.
Following are the therapeutic actions of benzodiazepines.

Action	Use
Anxiolytic	Anxiety disorders, alcohol withdrawal
Hypnotic	Premedication in anesthesia

Anticonvulsant	Sleep disorder
Muscle relaxant	Epilepsy, myoclonus, alcohol withdrawal
amnesic	Muscle spasticity and akathisia
Impairment of psychomotor function	Premedication

Commonly used Hypnotics

Clonazepam
Lorazepam
Midazolam
Flurazepam
Zolpidem
Zopiclone.

Adverse Effects of Benzodiazepines

1. Potential addiction forming tendency.
2. Sedation.
3. Risk of overdose.
4. Drowsiness and confusion.
5. Potentiate the effects of other CNS depressants
6. Orthostatic hypotension.
7. Nausea.

DRUGS FOR DEMENTIA (COGNITIVE ENHANCERS)

Drugs used in the management of dementia can be grouped as follows:

1. Cholinesterase inhibitors.
2. MMDA-Antagonists. (Glutamate Antagonist)
3. Non-steroidal-anti inflammatory drugs.
4. Vitamin C and E.
5. Psychotropic drugs.

Cholinesterase Inhibitors

1. Tacrine.
2. Metrifonate.
3. Donepezil.
4. Rivastigmine.
5. Galantamine.

Glutamate antagonist: Memantine.

It binds to the N-Methyl-D-Aspartate (NMDA) receptor operated cation channels, which activate glutamate. Glutamate is essential for learning and memory. Hence increasing his activity may improve learning and memory.

Psychotropic Drugs: Are useful in the dementia syndrome, where, severe demented patients exhibit cognitive behavioral and psychiatric symptoms. Low dose of antipsychotics like Quetiapine or low dose of antidepressants and low dose of mood stabilizers are preferred.

DRUGS USED TO TREAT EXTRAPYRAMIDAL SYNDROMES (EPS)

Anticholinergic agents closely resemble atropine with their ability to block muscarinic receptors and all are similar in action and efficacy for alleviating antipsychotic-induced EPS.

Common agents used to treat EPS

Category	Drug	Dose
Anticholinergic	Benztropine	0.5–6 mg
	Biperiden	2–6 mg
	Diphenhydramine	12.5–150 mg
	Procyclidine	2.5–22.5
	Trihexyphenidyl	1–15
Dopamine Facilitators	Amantadine	100–300
Beta-blockers	Propranolol	10–80
Alpha agonists	Clonidine	0.2–0.8

PSYCHOSTIMULANTS

Psychostimulants are nowadays indicated for the treatment of attention deficit hyperactive disorder (ADHD), narcolepsy, sleep apnea syndrome to reduce the excessive daytime sleepiness.

Following are some of the psychostimulants:

1. Amphetamines
2. Modafinil.
3. Atomoxetine.

Common Psychostimulants used to Treat ADHD

Drugs	*Dose mg/day*
D-amphetamine	5–40
Pemoline	37.5–112.5
Methylphenidate	10–60
Atomoxetine	40–100
Modafinil	100–200

These drugs are all somewhat different, but have the same basic effect. It may seem odd that stimulants can be used to control children who are hyperactive, the reason is the part of their brain that controls attention and impulsiveness is not working hard enough and needs to be stimulated.

Side effects of psychostimulants:
Headache, stomachache, sleepy and irritable behavior.

DRUGS FOR MANAGEMENT OF ALCOHOL DEPENDENCE

1. Disulfiram:
   Its main effect is to produce an unpleasant reaction in a person who drinks alcohol while he is on disulfiram treatment. Disulfiram interferes with the metabolism of alcohol by producing a marked increase in blood acetaldehyde levels. The accumulation of acetaldehyde produces unpleasant reaction called the disulfiram-alcohol reaction characterized by the following features:
   Nausea, throbbing headache, vomiting, hypotension, flushing, sweating, thirst, dyspnea, tachycardia, chest pain, vertigo, and blurred vision, occasionally because of the sudden fall in BP, patient may collapse.
   Dosage: Disulfiram 250 mg/day.
2. Acamprosate:
   This is a taurine derivative. It antagonizes glutamate, MMDA receptor function, it doubles the abstinent rates, reduces the relapse of alcohol abuse, it is an "anti-craving" drug.
   Dosage: Two 333 mg tablets (660 mg) taken three times a day.
3. Naltrexone:
   This is an opioid antagonist, in alcohol dependence, it reduces the relapse rate and reduces craving. It is contraindicated in acute hepatitis or liver failure.
   Dosage: 50–100 mg/day.
4. Topiramate: This anticonvulsant drug has recently been reported to improve drinking behavior. It is reported to reduce drinking days and increase the abstinence rate in alcohol dependence patients. It is given when the patient is still actively drinking.
   Dosage: 50–200 mg/day.

The three drugs namely, disulfiram, acamprosate and naltrexone should be initiated only after detoxification is over that is after the withdrawal symptoms is getting reduced.

Role of Nurse

The psychiatric nurse has a wealth of knowledge and techniques that make nursing unique in the care of the people with psychiatric disorders.

- Patient assessment
- Baseline information

- Prescribed psychiatric medication and nonpsychiatric medication
- Name of the drug
- Reason for taking
- Dates started and stopped
- Highest daily dose
- Who prescribed it
- Was it effective
- Side effects
- Coordination of treatment modalities
- Integrated in a holistic manner and
- Individualized for each patient.

Psychopharmacological drug administration
- Monitoring drug effects
- Medication education
- Drug maintenance programs
- Clinical research drug details
- Prescriptive authority.

SOMATIC THERAPIES (ELECTROCONVULSIVE THERAPY AND STIMULATION TECHNIQUES)

Electroconvulsive Therapy (ECT)

- Electroconvulsive therapy (ECT) is a procedure in which an electric current is applied across scalp electrodes to induce a grand mal seizure.
- ECT was introduced in 1938 in Italy by Cerletti and Bini.
- ECT is one of the time tested physical treatments in psychiatry, still in regular use, a fact that attests to its safety and efficacy.

ECT—Mode of Action

- The exact mode of action remains a mystery, yet, it is known to produce multiple effects on the CNS, including the down regulation of beta receptors commonly seen with antidepressants
- ECT has neuroprotective effects and stimulates neurogenesis. There is no evidence that ECT causes brain damage.

Indications for ECT

1. Major depressive disorder (Severe depression).
2. Bipolar disorder—Both in mania and depressive phase.
3. Schizophrenia—Especially in catatonic type.
4. Postpartum psychosis.
5. Depression during pregnancy.

ECT Procedure

Pretreatment Evaluation

a. Pertinent history of hypertension, musculoskeletal injuries, osteoporosis, recent myocardial infarction, bronchial asthma, seizures, and treatment with anticonvulsants and psychotropic drugs.
b. Preparing the patient—Informed consent, psychoeducation to patient and relatives, explaining the good and bad of ECT.

Procedure

A. Medications
   1. Anticholinergics—to minimize secretions (injection atropine).
   2. Anesthesia—Ketamine, propofol.
   3. Muscle relaxants—Succinyl choline.
B. Types of electrical stimuli
   1. Brief pulse.
   2. Sine wave.
C. Electrode placement
   1. Bilateral (Preferable).
   2. Unilateral (on non-dominated side of scalp).
D. Administering the stimulus
   1. Check the vital signs.
   2. Apply electrodes.
   3. Clear patient's mouth, remove any hearing aids, dentures.
   4. Begin anesthesia.
   5. Administer muscle relaxant.
   6. Ventilation.
   7. Apply bite block.
   8. Apply electrical stimulus.
   9. Induce a seizure that is therapeutic.
E. Monitoring
   1. ECG.
   2. EEG

ECT—Adverse Effects

1. Confusion.
2. Headache.
3. Nausea.
4. Muscle and joint pain.

5. Short-term amnesia.
6. Rarely prolonged apnea.
7. Mild cardiac arrhythmia.

Contraindications

1. Raised intracranial pressure.
2. Recent cerebrovascular accident.
3. Recent myocardial infarction.
4. Vascular aneurysm.
5. Retinal detachment.

Other Methods of Somatic Treatments

Other methods of somatic treatments are occasionally or rarely used in the treatment of resistant psychiatric disorders, they are:

1. Psychosurgery.
2. Transcranial magnetic stimulation (TMS).
3. Vagus nerve stimulation (VNS).
4. Sleep deprivation therapy.
5. Light therapy.

Psychosurgery

- Psychosurgery is the palliative neurosurgical procedure for refractory psychiatric disorders
- Major indication—chronic, debilitating, refractory mental disorders
- Cingulotomy, capsulotomy, subcaudate tractotomy, and limbic leucotomy are the main procedures used in psychosurgery
- Adverse effects of psychosurgery—apathy, seizures, memory impairment, incontinence, personality change, weight gain, disinhibition, and death
- Psychosurgery is not much practiced nowadays. To do psychosurgery, Mental Health Authorities approval and permission is essential.

Transcranial Magnetic Stimulation (TMS)

- Approved as a treatment method in psychiatry very recently
- Main indication is treatment resistant depression
- It involves the use of very short pulses of magnetic energy to stimulate nerve cells in the brain
- TMS produces focal secondary electrical stimulation of targeted cortical regions

- It is nonconvulsive. Requires no anesthesia and has a safe side effect profile
- TMS produces focal secondary electrical stimulation of targeted cortical regions
- It is nonconvulsive and requires no anesthesia and is not associated with cognitive side effects
- TMS is contraindicated in implanted metallic devices.

Vagus Nerve Stimulation (VNS)

- VNS therapy is a new modality of treatment method for a long time treatment resistant depression
- Its main indication is chronic or recurrent depression, which is resistant to routine antidepressant treatment
- Activation of the left vagus nerve has been shown to induce widespread bilateral effects in the brain including amygdala and the prefrontal cortex
- Common side effects of VNS—Temporary hoarseness of voice, increased coughing, shortness of breath on exertion and tickling of the throat.

PSYCHOLOGICAL METHODS OF TREATMENT

Treatment Methods in Psychiatry

In the management of mental health problems drugs alone cannot do the justice. The combination of drug treatment and psychological methods of treatment will be much more effective. The following are some of the methods by which psychologically we can understand the patient's problem and treat:

1. Psychoeducation and reassurance.
2. Counseling.
3. Psychotherapy
   a. Individual psychotherapy
   b. Group psychotherapy
   c. Family therapy
   d. Psychoanalysis.
4. Behavior therapy
   a. Systematic desensitization
   b. Flooding
   c. Modeling
   d. Response prevention
   e. Classical conditioning
   f. Operant conditioning

   g. Social skill training
   h. Aversion therapy and
   i. Cognitive behavior therapy
5. Relaxation therapy
6. Hypnotherapy (Hypnosis)
7. Biofeed back technique
8. Psychosocial rehabilitation.

Counseling

Counseling means understanding a person's problem and suggests various methods to cope up the situation. Counseling is different from psychotherapy. Counseling refers to professional assistance given to a variety of problems by discussion and advice. Counseling can be given to healthy individuals also and will not go into the depth of the problem or about the unconscious mental processes. A nurse, a doctor, a social worker, a teacher, a priest, a psychologist or a psychiatrist—any one of them can act as a counselor.

Characteristics of Good Counselor

- Genuine
- Sincere and concerned
- Empathic
- Nonjudgmental.

Psychotherapy

Psychotherapy is defined as the treatment of emotional disorders by psychological means. Its goal is to help people to cope better with life and achieve more emotionally satisfying lifestyles. Psychotherapy can help individuals to adapt to a new and challenging situation. Psychotherapy involves communication between two individuals. Psychotherapy involves many techniques which includes ventilation, abreaction, reassurance, suggestion, persuasion and relaxation. The following qualities are essential for a psychotherapist: He or she,

- Should understand the patients family and cultural background
- Should be a good listener
- Should have patience, sympathetic, understanding and tactful attitude
- Should have an interest and concern for the patients
- Should not be upset with patient's selfish and irresponsible behavior
- Should not be too emotionally involved with the patient and his problems
- Should not take sides and should act as nonjudgmental attitude.

Psychoanalytic Psychotherapy (Psychoanalysis)

Psychoanalysis is a form of psychotherapy, developed by the popular Austrian psychiatrist Sigmund Freud. It aims at uncovering conflicting, unconscious impulses through special techniques that include free association, dream analysis and transference.

In psychoanalysis, the therapist helps the patient to discover and cope with thoughts and feelings that direct his behavior but of which the patient is unaware.

Psychoanalytic psychotherapy is time-consuming and expensive. It may not be suitable for everyone.

Psychoanalysis is more commonly preferred in hysteria, other neurotic disorders and mild personality disorders. It is not suitable for psychosis.

Hypnotherapy (Hypnosis)

Hyposis is a psychophysiological, altered state of consciousness induced by conditioning and skilled use of suggestions.

It results in:

1. Lessening of the subjects inhibitions and reasoning.
2. Heightening of his ability to relax and his susceptibility to suggestion.

Hypnosis is an art based on science.

Steps of Hypnosis

a. Relaxation.
b. Realization of the cause of the problem.
c. Removal of the cause of the problem.
d. Rehabilitation.
e. Reinforcement (follow up).

Application of Hypnosis

1. In understanding the problem and conflicts which are deeply placed inside the mind.
2. In treating neurotic disorders especially hysteria, phobia and obsessive compulsive disorders, etc.
3. Without anesthesia, in the induction of labor and dental surgeries.
4. To alter unwanted behavior.
5. To teach self-hypnosis and to attain relaxation.
6. In the treatment of few psychosomatic disorders.

Hypnosis is not much practised by psychiatrists nowadays, it is an outdated practice, time consuming and not always reliable. Some of the psychotic disorders and personality disorders get aggravated after hypnosis.

BEHAVIOR THERAPY

Behavior therapy is based on the principles of learning theory. The therapy aims at modifying observable unwanted behavior. It is not bothered about unconscious thoughts or feelings. Various techniques are used to change the maladaptive behavior through changing the environmental influences. Two basic learning theories are;

I. Classical (Pavlovian) conditioning
II. Operant (Skinnerian) conditioning

- I. Classical conditioning
  - a. Systematic desensitization
  - b. Flooding
- II. Operant conditioning
  - a. Shaping
  - b. Chaining
  - c. Token economy
  - d. Aversion therapy.

COGNITIVE BEHAVIOR THERAPY (CBT)

CBT derives origins from psychoanalysis, cognitive psychology and behavioral psychology. CBT was developed by Beck in 1960 as a therapy for depression. CBT is a short-term therapy. Initally CBT evokes a lot of debate among clinicians. The cognitive triad consists of negative views regarding oneself, the world and the future. Cognitive errors are errors in thinking that maintain the negative schemes inspite of contradictory evidence. These lead to maladaptive behavior. In CBT, a therapist place active role and helps the patient to identify automatic thoughts, cognitive errors and maladaptive behaviors. Once identified, these faulty cognitions are challenged and substituted by alternative adaptive cognitions.

Relaxation Training

This is also known as Jacobson's progressive muscle relaxation training. The person is taught to tense up and then relax the major muscle groups of the body in a fixed order. By this training, patient learns to control the feeling of anxiety by relaxation. This works on the principle of reciprocal inhibition; that is anxiety and relaxation cannot coexist. This technique can be used alone to help persons with anxiety or pain (generalized anxiety disorder, low back pain, tension headache, etc.). The basic principle of relaxation training is: "relax your body, thereby relax your mind". Since, there is a strong relationsip between the mind and the body the relaxation of mind can be achieved through relaxation of the body muscles.

PSYCHOLOGICAL METHODS OF TREATMENT

Key Points

- Management of mental health problem requires not only drug treatment but also psychological methods of treatment
- Psychological treatment include:
  - Psychoeducation and reassurance
  - Counseling
  - Psychotherapy (Individual, group, family, psychoanalysis)
  - Behavior therapy (aversion therapy, systematic desensitition, operant conditioning, social skill training and cognitive therapy)
  - Relaxation therapy
  - Hypnotherapy
  - Biofeedback techniques
- Counseling means understanding a person's emotional problems and suggests methods to cop up the situation. Counseling may be often given married couples, students, addicts and persons with adjustment and emotional problem
- Psychotherapy is the treatment of emotional problems by psychological means; psychotherapy involves understanding the inner mind and analyzing the individual's personality techniques like ventilation, abreaction, reassurance, suggestion and persuasion.

  The therapist giving psychotherapy should be a sympathetic listener. He should have nonjudgmental attitude
- Psychoanalysis is based on the Freud's principle like free association, dream analysis and transference
- Behavior therapy is based on the principles of learning theory.

  It aims at modifying observable unwanted behavior. Unlearning the maladaptive behavior is the basic principle.

  The basic learning theories involved are:

  a. Classical (Pavlovian) conditioning

  b. Operant (Skinnerian) conditioning
- Cognitive behavior therapy is the popular model of behavior therapy in present day psychiatry

  Maladaptive behavior is due to negative cognition, which should be gradually eradicated by alternative adaptive cognition
- Hypnotherapy

  It is a psychophysicalogical altered state of consciousness induced by conditioning and skilled use of suggestion.

  Hypnosis is an art based on science.

  Relaxation removal of the symptoms or some of the basic steps.

ALTERNATIVE SYSTEM OF MEDICINE FOR TREATMENT OF MENTAL DISORDERS

1. Ayurveda
2. Yoga
3. Unani
4. Siddha
5. Homeopathy

Ayurveda

Ayurveda is an ancient Hindu system of medicine which originated in India. Ayurveda is based on the fact that illness is the result of falling out of balance with nature. Its diagnosis is based on three metabolic body types called as doshas. An ayurvedic doctor determines the dosha type as vata, pitta or kapha.

Treatment usually involves prescribing a diet, herbal remedies, , physical exercises, yoga meditation, massage and also by detoxification therapy.

Ayurveda is rapidly becoming more popular among people.

It incorporates an Individualized regimen—such as diet, meditation, herbal preparations, or other techniques—to treat a variety of conditions, including depression, to facilitate lifestyle changes, and to teach people how to release stress and tension through yoga or transcendental meditation.

Yoga

The tradition of Yoga was born in India several thousand years ago. Maharishi Patanjali is rightly called as the 'Father of Yoga.' Practitioners of this ancient Indian system of health care use breathing exercises, posture, stretches, and meditation to balance the body's energy centers. Yoga is used in combination with other treatment for depression, anxiety, and stress-related disorders.

Yoga discipline that focuses on the body musculature, posture, breathing mechanisms and consciousness.

Yoga is a method by which one can develop once inherent powers in a balanced manner. It offers the means to reach complete self-realizations. 'Yoga can be defined as a means for uniting the individual spirit with the universal spirit.'

Unani

Unani system of medicines originated in Greece and is based on the teachings of Hippocrates and Gallen and it developed into an elaborate

Medical System by Arabs, like Rhazes, Avicenna, Al-Zahravi, Ibne-Nafis and others.

Unani Tibb or Graeco—Arab medicine may be traced to that system of Greek medicine developed during the Arab civilization. Muslims still call it unani medicine but European historians call it Arab medicine. It is practiced in the Indo-Pakistan subcontinent.

The basic framework consists of four humor theory of Hippocrates, i.e. blood, phlegm, yellow bile and black bile. Temperament occupies a very important place in unani Tibb and forms a basis of pathology, diagnosis and treatment. Disease is an expression of the imbalance of the humors or the disturbance to their harmony.

Unani medicines got enriched by imbibing what was best in the contemporary systems of traditional medicines in Egypt, Syria, Iraq, Persia, India, China and other Middle East countries. In India, Unani system of medicine was introduced by Arabs and soon it took firm roots.

Unani system has shown remarkable results in curing the diseases like arthritis, leukoderma, jaundice, liver disorders, nervous system disorders, bronchial asthma, and several other acute and chronic diseases where other systems have not been able to give desired response. Now the system has crossed national boundaries and is popular among the masses globally.

Unani treatment is based on its natural and remarkable diagnosis methods and is affordable. It is mainly dependent on the temperament (Mizaj) of the patient, hereditary condition and effects, different complaints, signs and symptoms of the body, external observation, examination of the PULSE (Nubz), urine and stool, etc. Unique and special treatment methods like dietotherapy (Ilaj-bil-Ghiza), climatic therapy (Ilaj-bil-Hawa), regimental therapy (Ilaj-bit-Tadbir), make it a different and remarkable and popular system.

Siddha

Siddha system is one of the oldest systems of medicine in India. The term siddha means achievements and siddhas were saintly persons who achieved results in medicine. Eighteen siddhas were said to have contributed towards the development of this medical system. Siddha literature is in Tamil and it is practiced largely in Tamil-speaking part of India and abroad. The siddha system is largely therapeutic in nature. According to this system the human body is the replica of the Universe and so are the food and drugs irrespective of their origin.

This system believes that all objects in the Universe including human body are composed of five basic elements namely, earth, water, fire, air and sky. The food, which the human body takes and the drugs it uses are all, made of these five elements. The proportion of the elements present in the drugs vary and their preponderance or otherwise is responsible for certain actions and therapeutic results.

This system also deals with the concept of salvation in life. The exponents of this system consider achievement of this state is possible by medicines and meditation.

Homeopathy

Homeopathy, or homeopathic medicine, is a holistic system of treatment that originated in the late eighteenth century. The name homeopathy is derived from two Greek words that mean 'like disease.' The system is based on the idea that substances that produce symptoms of sickness in healthy people will have a curative effect when given in very dilute quantities to sick people who exhibit those same symptoms. Homeopathic remedies are believed to stimulate the body's own healing processes.

Homeopathy was founded by German physician Dr .Hahnemann (1755-1843), who was much disturbed by the medical system of his time, believing that its cures were crude and some of its strong drugs and treatments did more harm than good to patients. Hahnemann performed experiments on himself using Peruvian bark, which contains quinine, a *malaria* remedy. He concluded that in a healthy person, quinine creates the same symptoms as malaria, including fevers and chills, which is the reason why it is effective as a remedy. He then began to analyze the remedies available in nature by what he called proving. Proving of homeopathic remedies are still compiled by dosing healthy adults with various substances and documenting the results, in terms of the dose needed to produce the symptoms and the length of the dose's effectiveness. The proving are collected in large homeopathic references called Materia Medica or materials of medicine. This system of therapeutics helps to cure many mental disorders if a medicine is prescribed on the basis of individualized symptom analysis.

Chapter

25

Rehabilitation in Psychiatry

"Strength of mind is exercise, not rest"

—Alexander Pope, 18th Century Poet.

Rehabilitation in psychiatry is that process which attempts to benefit a mentally ill person back, as near as possible, to his original state. It is the process designed to help the handicapped individuals to make maximum use of their residual capacities and to enable them to lead a beneficial and meaningful life in the community.

Rehabilitation of the mentally ill, is an essential component of any therapeutic program that proposes to tackle effectively the maladies of mental illness. The proverb that' an idle mind is a devil's workshop' emphasizes the importance of activity in our day-to-day life. Activity may be physical, mental, social, and recreational or job oriented. In the case of mentally ill person due to various reasons, these activities are disturbed to a varying extent. Rehabilitation aims at helping the patient to re-establish or regain his interest to do useful activity.

The importance of psychological factors such as motivation, attitudes and personality in the rehabilitation process is well accepted. Rehabilitation is much beneficial to the long-term mentally ill people.

The following disorders are indicated commonly for rehabilitation.

1. Chronic schizophrenia
2. Chronic organic mental disorders
3. Mental retardation
4. Alcohol and drug dependence.

The goal of any treatment plan should be rehabilitation and reintegration of the patients to active community life. For successful rehabilitation co-operation of health care personnel, patients, their family members, opinion leaders and various voluntary agencies are indispensable.

Rehabilitation directs towards preparing the individual and his family to cope with a problem which is likely to persist for the rest of his life time. Considering the magnitude of the problem of mental morbidity in the country, the mental health professionals have a definite role to play in rehabilitation services for this group of people.

Rehabilitation involves training and educating the patient to deal more successfully with his problems.

OCCUPATION THERAPY

Occupation therapy is a rehabilitation process. Any activity, mental or physical which contributes to the recovery and rehabilitation of the mentally ill is known as occupation therapy in psychiatric setup.

Occupation therapy is an important part of therapeutic program. Persons who are trained to teach occupation therapy is known as occupation therapist. She or he will coordinate with doctors, nurses and social workers.

Aim

The aim is to provide a skilled program of daily activity for patients based on the knowledge of his personality, background habits, psychological problems and the diagnosis.

Advantages

Occupation therapy is helpful as a medium of treatment and as a medium of expression and communication. It helps the patients to engage in group activities, and they learn better along with other people. Occupation therapy improves the old skills, acquire new ones and reduce social isolation.

Occupation therapy provides many interesting and rewarding jobs for patients to do, some of them are:

1. Gardening
2. Painting
3. Carpentary
4. Needle and tailoring work
5. Mat weaving, basket making
6. Cooking
7. Secretarial work, etc.

Nurses Role

Nurses must spend some time during their training, in occupation therapy department. The experience they gain can be of great value in helping them to care for their patients. Nurses can assess their patients potentials, motivate them to attend OT and regularly supervise them whether they attend sincerely. They can encourage the patients who attend OT regularly by some incentives.

Occupational

- Prepare the patient for therapy
- Assist the therapist to administer therapies
- Take care of the patient after the therapies are over
- Find opportunity to give group and individual health education
- Keep link with the patients, families, and the therapist
- Coordinating the nursing service with psychosocial therapies.

INDUSTRIAL THERAPY

It is a part of rehabilitation process for the mentally ill. This puts work in its place as a part of rehabilitation. The patients aptitudes are related to simple commercial tasks and the work provided may be subcontracted out from industrial firms. The patient is paid according to his productivity. In this center, patients are specifically prepared for work in the community in full employment, or in a sheltered workshop.

Aims

1. Patients are encouraged to work and earn and to prepare them to live in the community in a useful way.
2. Recognizing the talents and interests of the mentally ill.
3. Imparting disciplines vocational training under sheltered condition.
4. Diverting the preoccupied mind to the performance of useful work.
5. Developing a certain degree of self-confidence and satisfaction through their economic independence.
6. Establishing a link between the mentally ill person and the society.

Following are some of the units run by certain centers.

1. Bakery unit.
2. Paper cover making unit.
3. Screen printing unit.
4. Toys and bags making unit.
5. Tailoring unit.
6. Soap unit.
7. Canteen.

RECREATIONAL THERAPY

Recreation is important for everyone, and not least for the patient in a psychiatric hospital. It provides interest and enjoyment and a welcome change from daily routine. Many patients have found it hard to enjoy social activities in the community often because difficulty in relating to other people. Social activities in hospital can help them to overcome their shyness and provide opportunities to develop personal relationship.

Recreational therapy must be carefully chosen to suit the needs of the individual patients, and should be given as much freedom of choice as possible. Elderly patients will often enjoy reading newspaper, listening to old time music, playing card, games, etc., younger patients will enjoy sports, games, music, etc., outings to places, 'interest, films, concerts and library facilities should be available everyone.

THERAPEUTIC COMMUNITY (THERAPEUTIC MILIEU)

The English psychiatrist Maxwell Jones, attempted to organize the psychiatric hospital as a therapeutic community. His primary goal is the elimination of the divisions between various mental health profession, which he believed to be artificial and harmful to the patient.

The milieu is everything that has impact upon the psychiatric inpatient. It is the manipulation of the patients environment in order to effect change in the behavior and personality of the individual.

The objectives of the therapy are:

1. Limit setting for the patient who is in need of it.
2. Learning the basic social skills of:
   a. Assertion
   b. Vocation
   c. Recreation.

The nurse should focus on patients problem solving methods and to motivate him for better rehabilitation. The important concept is that every mental health professional in a psychiatric hospital should understand and give due credit to the patient's right, privilege and responsibility to make decision about daily living activities in the treatment setting.

Characteristic of Milieu Therapy

1. A friendly, warm, trusting, secure, supportive comfort—atmosphere in the psychiatric ward.
2. An optimistic attitude about prognosis of the illness.
3. Better comforts, food and daily living needs for patients.
4. Better recognition to the patient and measures to improve his self-esteem. The nurse should call the patient by name and positively reinforce if he has done some good jobs.
5. Opportunity for patients to take responsibility in the day-to-day management of the wards including:
   a. Patient government
   b. Patient planned and patient directed social activities.

6. Opportunity to discuss interpersonal relationships in the unit among patients and patients and staff (decreased social distance between staff and patients).

ROLE OF A NURSE: TRIPARTITE ROLE

Authoritarian role: Controlling the group and setting limits.

Social role: Nurse encourages and support in various ways in communication discussion, and talking to the team members.

Therapeutic role: Effective therapeutic nurse-patient relationship.

Half-way Home

Advances in psychiatric treatment have made it possible to effectively control severe mental illness. With the discovery of effective therapies about 90 percent of today's mentally disturbed persons do not stay at hospitals for more than four to six weeks. Then it is possible to successfully reintegrate the majority of mentally disturbed persons back into society.

However even after treatment in hospitals, a small percentage who are severely mentally disturbed and emotionally sensitive, do not feel ready to cope with the outside world. Many of these people who do not require further hospitalization can be admitted as residents at the half-way home. The half-way home is a transition place that encourages constructive living and builds on resources and skills. It is therapeutic community and a home away from home and not a hospital. It is one of the big family with house parents, residents and staff interacting with each other with a family like closeness and a sense of belonging.

The half-way home is a place where each member is gradually trained to take up responsibilities under the guidance of caring professionals.

The residents are encouraged to modify them in appropriate behavior. They are involved in relearning, reconditioning and adjustment. This transformation takes place in the atmosphere of love and care provided at the half-way home. The prime objective of half-way home is to guide all residents towards self reliance. The activities of half-way home are directly supervised and conducted by a professional team consisting of Counselors/ social workers, occupational therapist, psychologist, house parents and consulting psychiatrists. Half-way homes are commonly run by voluntary agencies and missionaries.

Chapter 26

Psychiatric Emergencies

A psychiatric emergency is any disturbance in thoughts, feelings or actions for which immediate therapeutic intervention is necessary. It is any psychiatric condition or circumstance of a patient which calls for immediate action. Emergency in the psychiatric set up is usually due to one of the following reasons:

1. The patient may be a source of danger to himself or to others because of his mental state.
2. The patient's relatives may be extremely anxious regarding the patient's condition.
3. The patient may create disturbances in the community to an intolerant and unmanageable degree.
4. The patient may be in extreme and unbearable distress.

APPROACH TO A PSYCHIATRIC EMERGENCY

- Brief history to be taken,
- Assess the possibility of any probable precipitating factor
- Assess the distress and extreme behavior pattern
- Assess the degree of seriousness.

The Following Are the Common Psychiatric Emergencies

1. Excitement and violence.
2. Stupor.
3. Delirium.
4. Attempted suicide.
5. Panic attacks.
6. Epilepsy related emergencies.
7. Alcohol and other addictive drugs related psychiatric emergencies.
8. Antipsychotic drugs induced psychiatric emergencies.
9. Lithium toxicity.
10. Refusal of food.

ATTEMPTED SUICIDE

Any act of self-damage inflicted with self-destructive intention, however vague or ambivalent, is an attempted suicide.

If the patient dies as a result of the act it is called 'suicide', otherwise it is called attempted suicide.

A suicidal attempt with self-destructive intention is attempted suicide whereas an attempt without any intention of dying, but only to threaten or manipulate others, is called parasuicide or deliberate self-harm.

Attempted suicide is a cry for help. It is an act of despair. The ratio of attempted suicide to suicide is 10:1. Twenty percent of all admissions in medical emergency constitutes deliberate self-harm. The commonest age group which attempt suicide is 15–25 years. Females outnumber males in attempting suicide.

Evaluation of Attempted Suicide

It is advisable to get answers to the following questions to assess the suicidal patient.

1. Whether the patient belongs to the high-risk group?
    a. Old age, lonliness, social isolation.
    b. Mental illness—Severe depression, schizophrenia, hysteria, antisocial personality.
    c. Physical illness—Incurable, painful, long-term physical illness.
    d. Alcohol and drug dependence.
    e. Past history and family history of suicidal behavior.
2. The method used, Was it harmless or potentially fatal?
3. Is there any real intention to die? If so why?
4. The place and time, Was it carried out in the absence of others)?

Are there any serious risk factors?

5. Is there any significant recent loss, e.g. death of close relative, loss of job or self-esteem?
6. Were there any suicide talk, suicide letters, suicide plans?
7. Is there a will or any last wish? .

Management of Attempted Suicide

1. The initial intensive medical care of the acute physical conditions.
2. The psychological approach: Attempted suicide requires crisis intervention. Persons who attempt suicide need individual counseling and psychotherapy. Also, family and other significant people should be involved.

Nursing Care of Attempted Suicide

a. Give the patient an opportunity to express his feelings.
b. Improve communication by a sympathetic approach.
c. Strengthen self-esteem by supportive psychotherapy and reassurance.
d. Facilitate problem solving by:
   - identifying the problems,
   - identifying the alternatives,
   - being clear of the situation and practical solution,
   - choosing one alternative and following it up.

A person, who attempts suicide needs both medical and psychiatric treatment. The nurse must assess the severity of the injury. Medical resuscitation is the priority, only then psychiatric intervention is needed.

The patient's safety is a nursing priority. The nursing care starts with suicide prevention or preventing further attempts by making sure that the patient has no access to weapons, sharp objects, rope poisons, psychotropic drugs and situations where self harm can be inflicted. This requires close supervision by the nurse. Assessment and treatment, if underlying mental illness is present, is essential after the patient recovers from the critical condition.

Encourage verbalizations of honest feelings. Allow the patient to express angry feelings. Depression and suicidal behavior are viewed as anger turned inward on the self. If this anger can be verbalized the patient may become quiet, calm and comfortable.

The most important responsibility of the nurse is to spend some time with the person who attempted suicide. This provides a feeling of safety and security.

Crisis intervention is essential for the person who attempted suicide. This is more beneficial for persons who have interpersonal and marital problems. Crisis intervention is similar to supportive psychotherapy and includes ventilation abreaction and resolving conflicts. It starts with identifying the problems and ends with helping the person to understood and use non-suicidal methods to solve them.

Excitement (Violence)

Patients with excitement are prone for violence. They may harm others or harm themselves. Violence is physical aggression inflicted by one person on another. Violence may be done due to a wide range in psychiatric disorders.

Violence and threats of violence are frequently encountered in psychiatric emergency settings. The nurse should know how to rapidly initiate procedures for the prevention of violence.

Common Mental Disorders Associated with Excitement and Violent Behavior

1. Psychotic disorders
   a. Schizophrenia (especially paranoid and catatonic)
   b. Mania
   c. Paranoid disorders (delusional disorders)
   d. Postpartum psychosis.
2. Organic mental disorders
   a. Delirium
   b. Drug intoxication and withdrawal (alcohol and heroin)
3. Personality disorders
   a. Antisocial personality disorders
   b. Paranoid personality disorders
4. Brain disorders
   a. Seizure disorders (post-epileptic confusional state)
   b. Brain injury, encephalitis
   c. Mental retardation with behavior problem.

Following are some important questions a nurse should ask a relative or the person accompanying an excited patient to have quick assessment:

1. Is the person a known mentally ill? If so what type and what treatment has he been taking?
2. Has he had a similar excitement earlier?
3. Is there any history of loss of consciousness, head injury epilepsy, alcoholism or drug addiction?
4. Is he involved in any criminal or antisocial activity?

Nursing Care of a Violent and Excited Patient

1. First protect yourself, do not approach alone, call for assistance to manage any situation. Do not close the door of the consulting room. Leave physical restraint to the staff members who are trained for that.
   - Do not challenge or confront a violent patient
   - Always keep an eye of a way through which you can escape
   - Never turn your back on the patient
   - Be sure that sufficient staff members are there to restrain the patient.
2. After physical restraint, approach the patient cautiously; do not be too brave or confident.
3. The most effective drugs are:
   - Injection Chlorpromazine 100 mg IM
   - Injection Haloperidol 10–20 mg IM/IV
   - Injection Diazepam 10 mg IV (slowly).

   If there is a history of head injury or brain infection avoid these drug;

4. Assess the nutritional state and, if there is dehydration, IV fluid are essential.
5. Attend to the external injury, if required.
6. If psychiatric treatment is not needed you may call the police for help.

Stupor

Stupor is a condition where the patient is conscious, but there is non-responsiveness to the surroundings. There will be total absence of self care, neglecting physiological needs like food and fluid intake and almost total motor inactivity. Stupor can occur in two mental disorders.

1. Schizophrenia (especially catatonic)
2. Depression.

These are emergencies because there is risk of neglect with the nutritional needs of the body.

Nursing Care

Assess the nutritional states and hydration. Give immediate VI fluids and ryles tube feeding, if necessary. Plenty of vitamins are also essential as well as physiotherapy to facilitate movements and to prevent contractures. Minimal dose of drugs (antipsychotics or antidepressants) are helpful to relieve basic problems.

DELIRIUM

Delirium is an acute organic mental disorder. It is a sign of acute brain dysfunction and is therefore an emergency. The important clinical factors of delirium are: confusion, clouding of consciousness disorientation, insomnia, nightmares, illusions and hallucinations restlessness, perplexity, agitated mood, increased autonomic system activity, fever and fits. The patient is more disturbed during the night.

Delirium is often reversible, the course usually being brief and fluctuating. Delirium is common in the medically ill, hence most often seen in a general hospital setting. It is commonly seen in medical wards, surgical wards, trauma wards, geriatric wards and deaddiction wards.

Important Causes of Delirium

1. Severe infections—Typhoid, pneumonia, septicemia, puerperal sepsis.
2. Intracranial infections—Encephalitis, meningitis, cerebral malaria, cerebral abscess.
3. Acute brain disorders—Head injury, cerebral hemorrhage, hypertensive encephalopathy.

4. Metabolic disturbance—Uremia, liver failure, cardiac failure, respiratory failure, electrolyte imbalance.
5. Vitamin deficiency—Pellagra (nicotinamide) Wernicke's encephalopathy (thiamine).
6. Drug withdrawal—From opiates (heroin), alcohol (delirium tremens), barbiturates.
7. Drug intoxication—Atropine, cocaine, bromide.

Nursing Management of Patients with Delirium

- Keep the patient in a well ventilated room with good lighting
- Assess the vital signs periodically
- Assess the hydration and level of consciousness
- Watch for an attack of fit or altered behavior
- Identify any likely cause from the history of the patient
- Remember that if untreated, delirium can lead to death
- If the patient is agitated, physical restraint may be necessary
- Correct any metabolic, nutritional, electrolyte or fluid imbalance
- Fever and fit to be treated appropriately
- Start the treatment when a definite diagnosis is made.

Injection haloperidol 2–5 mg is helpful when the patient is agitated and restless. If it is alcohol or drug withdrawal delirium or associated fit is there, Injection diazepam 10 mg slow IV may be helpful; gradually oral treatment with anti-psychotics or benzodiazepines may be continued. Associated infections should be treated with appropriate antibiotics.

PANIC ATTACK (PANIC DISORDERS)

Panic attack is a severe form of acute anxiety. Panic disorder is characterized by spontaneous, episodic and intense periods of anxiety. It usually lasts for few a minutes to 30 minutes. Panic disorders usually occur once or twice a week.

The symptoms of panic disorder include:

- Shortness of breath (dyspnea)
- Dizziness, feeling unsteady or faint
- Palpitations (tachycardia)
- Trembling or shaking
- Increased sweating
- Choking sensations
- Abdominal distress
- Flushes or chills
- Chest pain or discomfort (without any ECG abnormality)

- Fear of dying
- Fear of going crazy
- Not all the above symptoms should occur to call it a panic attack; just four or more symptoms may be sufficient. In the typical case, the patient has been repeatedly presented to the emergency rooms or a doctor's consulting room, with physical symptoms, feelings of uneasiness, chest pain, fear of dying, etc.
- All the above symptoms occur despite the absence of cardiac or medical disease. Panic attacks can be provoked by inhalation of carbon dioxide (CO_2), psychosocial stressor may also precipitate an attack of panic. Most of these patients suffer from anticipatory anxiety.

Management and Nursing Care

It is very essential to map out all possible causes for panic symptoms. All the necessary investigations, especially ECG, should be taken. It is necessary to get a detailed history about the patient's, medication and drugs.

Management of panic disorder includes drug treatment behavior therapy, supportive psychotherapy and relaxation therapy.

The drugs commonly used in the management of panic attacks are:

1. Alprazolam (Alzolam, Anxit, Restyl, etc.) 0.25–05 mg every hours.
2. Lorazepam (Ativan, Larpose, etc.) 1–2 mg every 4 hours.
3. Clonazepam (Rivotril, Lonazep, etc.) 0.5–2 mg.

Sometime even higher doses may be required to control panic attacks. Tricylic antidepressants like Imipramine are also effective. If the attack is very severe Injection diazepam one ampule IV slowly may be useful in rare case.

The nursing care of panic disorders include the following measures:

1. It is essential to explain the nature of the disease to the patient, i.e. it is only an acute form of anxiety, and an emotional problem. There is no risk to her life, and things will settle down totally after proper treatment. This sort of health education to the patient and to the relatives will provide insight regarding this dreadful disease. This sort of reassurance itself will dramatically improve the situation.
2. Sometimes panic disorder patients are uncooperative to the nurse. They are tense, trembling, sweating and feel faint. The nurse should act in a calm and quiet manner to handle such patients.
3. Medication like oral alprazolam, clonazepam or lorazepam or, occasionally injection diazepam as instructed should be administered.
4. It is important to teach the patient to reduce their coffee and alcohol intake and smoking. Caffine, alcohol and nicotine are potentially anxiety producing chemicals.

Epilepsy Related psychiatric Emergencies

There are two conditions related to epilepsy which are to be considered as emergencies.

1. Status epilepticus
2. Postictal (epileptic) confusional state.

In status epilepticus, seizures follow one another with no intervening periods of consciousness. The seizures may be fatal. They may produce cerebral anoxia (poor oxygen supply to the brain) and hence cause brain damage. The patient should be immediately hospitalized. IV fluids, oxygen, IV diazepam (very slowly) or parenteral phenytoin are the emergency measures to be adopted.

In the postictal confusional state the patient may become excited, violent and may harm himself or others. Immediate physical restraint, injection diazepam IV and, if necessary, injection haloperidol IV are the first steps. The patient is usually confused and will be amnesic of the confusional period.

Alcohol and Other Addiction Forming Drugs and Psychiatric Emergencies

The common emergencies under this are:

1. Alcohol intoxication (pathological intoxication)
2. Acute alcoholic withdrawal state (delirium tremens)
3. Alcohol overdose (poisoning)
4. Disulfiram—alcohol reaction
5. Opioid intoxication and withdrawal.

Alcohol Intoxication

Its also called pathological intoxication. It is maladaptive behavior, usually aggressive (e.g. fighting) that occurs after consuming alcohol. The condition is associated with slurred speech, uncoordinated, unsteady gait, nystagmus and flushed face.

The management aims to help the patient through intoxication without injury to self or others. When the patient becomes sober, educate him to undergo deaddiction treatment. If the patient is violent or agitated injection haloperidol 5–10 mg or injection lorazepam 2 mg by mouth can be given.

Alcohol Withdrawal Delirium (DT or Delirium Tremens)

This is a severe complication of alcohol withdrawal that occurs in about five percent of patients withdrawing from alcohol. This condition is potentially life-threatening, if untreated. Delirium tremens cases are commonly seen in deaddiction wards, trauma care units (accidents due to drunken driving), postoperative wards and in gastroenterology clinics where patients with alcohol dependence get treatment for alcohol related disorders.

The management of DT requires treatment in the intensive medical care unit. Dehydration and electrolyte imbalance should be corrected by IV fluids. Associated medical problems like head trauma, rib fracture, infection, gastrointestinal bleeding and liver disease should be attended to. Keep a watch for any neurological deficit. Sometimes withdrawal fit (rum fit) may occur which should be symptomatically treated with IV diazepam.

Nursing care includes careful monitoring of vital signs, watching for any physical or psychological complications. Avoid physical restraint. Keep the patient in a quiet, calm environment. There should be good lighting in the room. Administer vitamins especially B1 (Thiamine) 100 mg IM. Carry out the instructions of the doctor regarding medications like injection diazepam or chlordiazepoxide to control withdrawal symptoms and fits, liver preparations, IV fluids, vitamins, etc.

Alcohol Overdose (Poisoning)

It is the ingestion of a quantity of alcohol sufficient to cause severe toxicity, coma or death.

A blood level of 0.1 to 0.15 percent alcohol indicates intoxication, a level of 0.3 to 0.4 percent usually induces coma and higher level may cause death. Death may be due to respiratory depression or the aspiration of vomitus.

Alcohol overdose can occur in two conditions:

1. As a suicide attempt.
2. As an accident.

Prompt medical attention is essential. Gastric lavage, intubation and care in an intensive medical care unit is essential. Administer 25 or 10 percent dextrose and oxygen immediately, and then depending upon the complications, follow the doctor's advice.

Disulfiram Alcohol Reaction

This may occur in patients who are undergoing alcohol deaddiction treatment with disulfiram (Antabuse, Esperal). When the patient is on this drug, if he consumes alcohol it may produce a severe reaction which sometimes becomes fatal due to a sudden fall in BP. When a patient is on disulfiram treatment if he is found unconscious, it may be due to this reaction. The patient should be immediately hospitalized. IV fluids, injection dexamathasone, dopamine drip (if needed) injection avil and oxygen should be given immediately.

Opioid Intoxication and Withdrawal

Opioid intoxication follows the recent ingestion, inhalation or injection of an opioid preparation. It is characterized by drowsiness, euphoria, analgesia, slurred speech, impaired attention, loss of appetite, etc. Opioid intoxication can lead to opioid overdose, which can be a life-threatening emergency. The opium drugs (including synthetic) are opium, morphine, heroin (brown sugar), methadone, codeine, pentazocine (fortwin), buprenorphine (tidigesic) and propoxyphene (proxyvon), pethidine, etc.

Management of opioid intoxication requires assessment of vital signs, a detailed history about drug behavior and assessing other medical problems like hepatitis, AIDS, thrombophlebitis, cardiac and respiratory disorders.

If CNS depression or respiratory depression is there, it indicates overdose. Treat with naloxone 0.8 mg IV, if no improvement after 15 minutes gives another 1.6 mg IV. It can be repeated later depending upon the need. Ask the patient to undergo a deaddiction treatment program.

Opioid withdrawal (like heroin withdrawal) occurs after the cessation or decrease in the dose of opioids taken by a long-term, user. The withdrawal symptoms are called by the user as 'Turky'. The features are craving for the drug, pupillary dilation, piloerection, sweating, fever, insomnia, yawning, nausea, vomiting, severe body and abdominal pain and rhinorrhea and diarrhea. The patient will be agitated, restless, irritable, quarrelsome and violent. They may harm themselves or others.

To obtain the drug and to reduce the painful withdrawal symptoms they may indulge in antisocial activity like fighting stealing, robbery, etc.

The management includes admission of the patient in deaddiction ward. Administration of IV fluids, antianxiety drug like chloridiazepoxide or diazepam, painkillers like ibuprofen antispasmodics and antidiarrheals. Administer methadone 10 mg by mouth every four hours. Methadone is the primary long-term treatment for opioid dependence. Naltrexone, a long-acting opioid antagonist, can be given orally for up to 2 months to help patient, maintain their abstinence from opioids. Clonidine 0.1 to 0.2 mg every three hours may relieve some of the patient's withdrawal symptoms like nausea, vomiting and diarrhea.

Antipsychotic Drugs Induced Emergency—Acute Dystonia

It is the slow involuntary contraction of one or more muscle group. Acute dystonia can occur following the administration of antipsychotic drugs in some patients, in one or two day's time. It consists of stiffness of the neck, mouth and tongue and elevation of the eye ball.

Dystonia produces discomfort to the patient and it is frightening relative. Dystonia is an extrapyramidal side-effect. Acute Dystonia can be relieved by injection promethazine (phenergan) or benadryl syrup by mouth. Dystonia can usually be prevented by the prophylactic use of Antiparkinsonian drugs like trihexy-phenidyl (Pacitane).

Lithium Toxicity

It is a psychiatric emergency. It is produced by an excess of lithium. The toxic state affects the central nervous system, thyroid, kidneys gastrointestinal system and metabolic system. Lithium levels are increased by dehydration, low salt intake, decreased fluid intake and many non-steroidal anti-inflammatory drugs. The optimum serum lithium level is 0.8 to 1.5 mmol/L. The serum lithium level above 2.0 mmol/L is toxic. The toxic effects are tremor, diarrhea, vomiting, drowsiness, unsteadiness and fit.

Management of Lithium Toxicity

Before administering lithium to a patient certain important investigations like complete blood count, blood urea, creatinine, thyroid functions and ECG are essential.

The treatment of lithium toxicity includes abrupt stopping of lithium. IV normal saline and diuretics (Injection lasix). Hemodialysis is very effective in reaching the normal serum lithium levels. Other cardiac complications are to be attended to.

The important nursing care is the periodic serum lithium assessment and having the patient take plenty of water along with the treatment. If any signs of toxicity appear (which the patient should be aware of) he should report them immediately.

Refusal of Food

Psychiatric patients may at times refuse to take food. It may be due to the following reasons:

1. They are not bothered about their nutrition (schizophrenia).
2. Suspect that their food is poisoned (paranoid disorders).
3. Loss of appetite, lack of interest (depression).
4. Too busy and active that they do not have time to eat (manic patient).
5. As a suicidal gesture (depression).
6. As a protest against the hospitalization, treatment or an attention-seeking behavior (antisocial personality disorder and drug addiction).
7. Associated with other physical illnesses (like tuberculosis).

Hence, it is essential for a nurse to supervise the diet regularly and see that the patient takes adequate food. Sometimes a greedy, much too hungry or hyperactive patient may take away the food of a dull, withdrawn or mentally retarded one. Hence, these patients will not get their food and starve. Sometimes, due to physical illness like fever, diarrhea (which they cannot express due to their subnormal intelligence or withdrawn behavior), they may not eat properly. It is the duty or the nurse to be aware of all these situations.

Regular diet supervision and maintenance of the weight chart are essential duties of a nurse in a psychiatric ward. The nurse should encourage and support patients with problems, motivate the withdrawn ones and train the mentally retarded children to eat properly. Sometimes, in acute cases, it may be necessary to give IV fluids or ryle's tube feeding. General hospital patients are mostly looked after by relatives but chronic patients in the mental hospital set up mostly depend upon the hospital diet.

Diet supervision and effective management of refusal of food are therefore essential duties of a nurse in a psychiatric hospital.

Chapter

27

Mental Health Nursing Care in Specific Situations

NURSING CARE OF A VIOLENT PATIENT

Violence is physical aggression inflicted by one person on another. Violence can be due to a wide range of psychiatric disorders, but it may also occur in normal people. Violence and threats of violence are frequently encountered in psychiatric emergency settings.

Violence can occur in the following psychiatric disorders:

1. Psychiatric disorders.
   - Schizophrenia especially paranoid or catatonic
   - Mania
   - Paranoid disorders (delusional disorders)
   - postpartum psychosis
   - Organic mental disorders.
2. Delirium
   - Drug intoxication or withdrawal
   - Antisocial (psychopathic) personality disorder.
3. Seizure disorder—postictal confusional state.
4. Mental retardation with behavioral problem.

Nursing Responsibility

The basic objective is to protect self and the patient. Never confront or argue a patient who is violent. Never interview an armed patient. Never be alone with a violent patient. Keep enough staff members with you. Call for staff assistance before the patient's agitation increases.

Physical restraint of patients may be necessary to prevent violence. Physical restraint is an important, useful and often necessary intervention. Leave physical restraint to those who are specifically trained for it. Once the patient is restrained, offer medication depending upon the disorder suspected. Injection chlorpromazine (Largactil) 50–100 mg, deep in the gluteal region, injection haloperidol 20 mg IM/IV or Injection diazepam 10 mg IV (slow) are the drugs of choice in managing violent patients.

Continue to monitor the patient's vital signs every half-an-hour, while the patient is in restraint. IV fluids are essential because of possible exhaustion and dehydration. Watch for any physical injury and attend to that. Document the findings, medication given and reasons for placing the patient in restraint.

If any family member, relative or friend of the patient is nearby quickly assess the cause for violence. Ask the following:

1. Was there any previous attack of similar violence?
2. Is the patient suffering from any psychiatric disorder and is he getting treatment for it?
3. Is the person an alcoholic or drug abuser?
4. Is there any recent history of injury (especially head injury) infection or intoxication?

These are all some basic questions which may give a clue to the underlying disorder. Hospitalization may be necessary to detain the patient and to prevent violence. Constant observation of a patient's behavior and his fluid and food intake is essential.

It is very important that a nurse working in a psychiatric emergency setting should able to recognize the high risk patients and act immediately.

NURSING CARE OF A WITHDRAWN PATIENT

In a clinical psychiatric setting, some patients are dull and withdrawn. At one end, their activity will be less and at the other end they will be stuporous.

The associated features are: negativism, lack of communication, posturing, refusal of food, not having initiation and motivation with loss of energy. This withdrawn state may occur in the following psychiatric conditions:

1. Chronic schizophrenia.
2. Catatonic schizophrenia.
3. Depression.
4. Some cases of dementia.
5. Long-term cannabis (ganja) abuse.
6. Long-term stay in mental hospitals (institutional neurosis).

Nursing Responsibility

It includes taking care of:

1. Physical needs.
2. Emotional needs.
3. Maintaining a therapeutic environment.

Meeting Physical Needs

1. Withdrawn patients are prone to many physical problems. Maintaining good personal hygiene and a planned routine will contribute towards improving general health.
2. Diet should be related to the degree of activity shown. The patient may have to be fed if he becomes too preoccupied to eat.
3. Elimination has to be carefully watched. The patient should be taken to the toilet at regular intervals.
4. Faulty circulation would result when a patient seldom moves. Even contractures may occur if a patient is too withdrawn and/or a long period. His position should be changed at least every two hours, clenched hands should be opened and a ball of gauze or cotton inserted at various times during the day.

Meeting Emotional Needs

1. The withdrawn patient is shy, sensitive and distrustful of relationship because persons associated with him during childhood were cold, distant and unable to give the warm, loving care needed for mature emotional development. Hence, these patients have problems in relationships, particularly with family members. They can be best helped by warmth, sincerity and honesty. You must take the initiative in establishing a positive relationship with him (feelings of trust and confidence).
2. The patient must be kept in contact with reality though he may resist. The patient does have a degree of awareness. What you say to him and how you care for him can induce interest and give hope. Do not look for immediate success.
3. Maintain a warm, positive and respectful attitude towards the patient, so that he begins to feel secure in his relationships. A person is able to give love only if he has received love. Respecting the patient as a person is important. He should be addressed by his correct name and treated with dignity.
4. The delusions and hallucinations of the patient should never be made the subject of ridicule. Do not argue and contradict his statements. Give short and honest replies.

Maintaining a Therapeutic Environment

1. These patients should be encouraged to have walking and group games.
2. Sometimes the patient may ridicule the nurse or make some sarcastic comments. The nurse should develop a tolerance for this behavior.
3. For the patients who need stimulation, occupational and recreational therapies should be provided. Emphasis is placed on reassurance, readjustment, reeducation and rehabilitation.

4. Group therapy may promote socialization.
5. The nurse can play an important role in preventing the patient's retreat from reality by providing surroundings and contacts that are so pleasant and non-threatening that he will want to accept and enjoy them.

NURSING CARE OF ACCIDENT PRONE MENTALLY ILL

Persons suffering from mental illnesses are more accident prone.

The reasons are:

1. They are not aware of the common dangers.
2. They are preoccupied; some of them at times are in a dreamy state.
3. Some mentally ill are confused, some may be excited and find it difficult to stay in one place.
4. Under intoxication, some persons may have unsteady walk and often fall down.
5. Some may fall down in an altered state of consciousness and injure themselves.
6. Some deliberately harm themselves.
   - Persons suffering from mental retardation are unable to understand the common dangers and are prone to get involved in accidents, e.g. they may cross the road without noticing the traffic or go near the fire and injure themselves
   - Similarly, persons suffering from dementia, because of their deteriorating mental capacities and poor judgment, are likely to be involved in accidents
   - Persons suffering from major mental disorders like schizophrenia are often preoccupied, live in their fantasy world or act upon to the influence of delusions and hallucinations. They are prone to get injured in accidents as they wander aimlessly
   - Persons suffering from delirium are often confused, agitated and have increased psychomotor activity. Because of this, they may get injured
   - Persons suffering from manic excitement and schizophrenia are also prone to get involved in accident
   - Children suffering from ADHD (attention deficit hyperactive disorder) are hyperactive and are highly accident prone and get injured often
   - Persons who drink alcohol excessively and have unsteady gait and uncontrolled behavior are prone to get into accident. People who drive under the influence of alcohol (drunken driving) have a high risk of accidents
   - Persons suffering from epilepsy fall down during an attack unconsciously and get injured. In the same way, persons suffering

from organic mental disorders may also fall down in an altered conscious state and get injured

- Persons suffering from hysteria or from depression may sometimes deliberately harm themselves. Some attempts suicide and in this process get injured
- Nurses who work with the mentally ill, should know all these conditions where the risk of accident is high. The following are some steps to minimize accidents and injuries:
  1. Sharp objects are to be avoided where children with mental retardation, hyperactive people and persons with dementia move around.
  2. Health education regarding the ill effects of alcoholism, the dangerousness of drunken driving should be given.
  3. Persons suffering from psychosis should be adequately treated. Those who are accident prone should be kept under safe custody.
  4. Sometimes people suffering from delirium should be physically restrained.
  5. Epileptics are advised not to go near fire, moving machines and swimming pools. When a person gets a fit, see that no sharp objects are around the place.
  6. Persons who have ideas of suicide and deliberate self harm should be recognized earlier and effectively treated. Counseling and supportive psychotherapy and crisis intervention have to be carried out.
  7. Educating the care givers, especially the family members regarding the accident proneness in these individuals and also instructing them how to provide a safe environment is very important.
  8. Sometimes patients who are on psychotropic drugs may be drowsy and may fall down or get injured in accidents. Hence, persons who are on active treatment should be advised rest and not allowed to work with machinery and drive vehicles.
  9. The nurses motto should be 'Patient's safety is a nursing priority'. when working with the mentally ill.

NURSING CARE OF SUICIDAL PATIENT

Suicide is intentional self-inflicted death. Suicidal ideation, gesture and attempted suicide are the most common psychiatric emergencies. A suicide attempt is an act of self damage. If the patient dies as a result of the act it is called suicide otherwise the act is called attempted suicide.

Common objectives of a suicide include:

1. A crisis that causes intense suffering and feelings of hopelessness and helplessness.
2. Conflict between survival and unbearable stress (ambivalence to die or to live).
3. A wish to escape from reality.

Identifying a suicidal patient is a crucial but difficult task. Males of advancing age and social isolation have an increased risk of completed suicide. Young females, neurotics and people unable to cope with stress have increased risk of attempted suicide. Brief interview and evaluation of a suicidal patient is essential. At the end of the assessment, the nurse should be in a position to answer the following questions.

1. Whether the person belongs to high risk group?
   - Old age, loneliness, social isolation, male
   - Mental illness—severe depression, schizophrenia, antisocial personality disorder
   - Chronic, painful, intractable physical illness, e.g. cancer
   - Past history and family history of sucidial behavior.
2. The method used, was it harmless or potentially fatal?
3. If the intention to die is real and severe?
4. The place and time—If the act is carried out early in the morning, in the absence of others, it indicates severe intention to die.
5. If there is a significant recent loss, e.g. death of a close relative, loss of job or prestige.
6. If there have been any failure in the recent past, e.g. failure in exams, love.
7. If there is any last preparation—suicide notes, letter, will, etc.

Nursing Responsibility

The nurse should understand that a person is attempting suicide:

1. Because of desperation or hopelessness or
2. To manipulate the environment or
3. As an attention seeking behavior.

A suicide attempt is cry for help. Such people are undergoing emotional crisis or turmoil and what they want is an opportunity to ventilate their emotion. It is like doing an incision and drainage (1 and 0) of an abscess, to let out the pus, thereby relieving the pain, In a psychological crisis, emotional ventilation gives relief to the intense suffering and torture. This is the aim of the crisis intervention therapy.

When evaluating suicidal patients do not leave them alone, remove any potentially dangerous objects (e.g. knife, scissors, razor, etc.) from the vicinity make sure that the patient is swallowing the medication you give; the suicidal patient sometimes stores the drugs, to swallow later in an attempt to commit suicide.

In the emergency ward and in the psychiatric ward, the nurse has to be particularly vigilant.

After initial emergency medical treatment, the treatment for the underlying mental disease should be continued. For other marital and social problem, the other significant people are to be involved in the psychotherapy. Crisis intervention is a form of psychotherapy which includes ventilation, abreation and resolving the conflict. It starts with identifying the problems and ends with helping the patient to understand and use nonsuicidal methods to solve them.

NURSING CARE OF PATIENTS WITH DELUSIONS (PARANOID PATIENTS)

Delusions are false, fixed beliefs, out of proportion to reality, and cannot be removed by reason or logic. In paranoid delusion, for example, the person believes that he is the subject of persecution and people are looking at him, talking about him and plotting against him. He may regard a parked car as suspicious and believe that the people inside the car are policemen following him.

Patients with delusions are preoccupied with them and they react to the delusion. Their whole behavior pattern is centered around their delusional system

Delusions commonly occur in the following conditions:

1. Schizophrenia (especially paranoid schizophrenia).
2. Delusional disorders (all delusions).
3. Mood disorders—depression, mania.
4. Organic mental disorders—delirium, dementia.
5. Alcohol dependence and ganja dependence.

NURSING CARE OF DELUDED PATIENTS

Persons with predominant delusions (paranoid) are irritable and hostile.

When a nurse comes across a patient with a false belief, it is advisable not to argue or confront with him. Try to understand his delusion, his background and confirm it with relatives. After initial treatment with antipsychotic drugs and/or ECT, try to make him understand that his belief may not be true also.

Patients with delusions are suspicious, irritable and aggressive, suddenly they become violent. So the nurse should keep some assistants along with her. If necessary physical restraint may be requested before starting interview or treatment.

Patients with delusions often feel that their food is being poisoned and drugs will kill him. This refusal of food should be tackled carefully by supervising his diet or, if necessary, giving IV fluids and tube feeding. In the initial period of treatment antipsychotic drugs like haloperidol or chlorpromazine should be given in injection forms.

Deluded patients are highly impulsive. They are hostile. If hostility is directed towards others it ends in violence and homicide (murder) and if the hostility is directed towards self they may harm themselves (suicide).

Depressed patients who have delusions of nihilism feel that they are hopeless, helpless and the whole world is coming to an end, hence based on their delusional thinking, they may harm themselves. This suicidal idea should be identified and treated accordingly.

In some patients, delusions may be encapsulated; hence treatment may not have any effect on his delusion, and he may be without any active problem.

NURSING CARE OF THE AIDS PATIENT

Acquired immunodeficiency syndrome (AIDS) is a disease, at least moderately predictive of a defect in cell mediated immunity, occurring in a person with no known cause for a diminished resistance to that disease. AIDS, as a clinical condition, was first described in 1981. The human immunodeficiency virus (HIV) is transmitted through infected bodily fluids, in particular semen and blood. AIDS is lethal and has reached epidemic proportions.

The high-risk group includes

1. Persons having multiple sexual partners of high-risk group and do not adhere to safe sex practices.
2. Male homosexuals.
3. Intravenous drug users.
4. Recipients of blood transfusions.
5. Persons with open wounds that were exposed to HIV contaminated blood.

NEUROPSYCHIATRIC COMPLICATIONS OF AIDS

Functional psychiatric disorders

- Depression
- Anxiety disorders
- Adjustment disorders
- Psychosis.

Organic mental disorders
- Delirium
- Dementia (AIDS dementia complex)
- Organic personality disorders.

Neurological disorders
- CNS metastasis of Kaposi's sarcoma
- Primary CNS lymphoma
- Opportunistic CNS infection such as toxoplasmosis, herpes, etc.
- Seizures.

NURSING CARE OF AIDS PATIENTS

When treating a known or suspected HIV positive patient, protect staff members, family members and other patients from possible exposure. Nurses who care for these patients should take proper precautions. Mild adjustment disorders, anxiety disorders and depression can generally be treated with brief supportive psychotherapy.

The general approach is similar to that used with cancer patients. Working through guilt feelings about high-risk behavior is often important. Talking about safe sexual practices and the cessation of IV drug abuse should be the priority.

COUNSELING

- Pre-test HIV Counseling
- Discuss the meaning of a positive result (the test detects exposure to the AIDS virus; it is not a test for AIDS)
- Discuss the meaning of a negative result (Seroconversion requires time, recent high-risk behavior require follow up testing)
- Be available to discuss the patient's fears and concerns
- Discuss why the test is necessary
- Explore the patients potential reactions to a positive result (e.g. "I will kill myself if I am positive"). Take appropriate steps to intervene in such reactions
- Discuss the confidentiality issue
- Discuss how a seropositive result can affect social status
- Explore the high-risk behavior and recommend risk reducing interventions
- Document discussions in the patient's chart
- Allow the patient to ask questions.

Post-Test HIV Counseling

- Interpretation of test results should be done carefully and tactfully
- Guide him to prevent transmission to sexual partners and needle contacts
- If the test result is positive, tell him to avoid donating blood and organs. Ask him to keep separate razors and toothbrushes
- Be part of the mental health team to support the patient and his emotional problems like guilt, depression, fear of death, etc.
- Encourage family members and community services to support the patients.

NURSING CARE OF DYING PATIENTS

Death is not simply a biological event, it involves a complex psychological process also. The process of death has had frightening aspects. The attitude towards death and dying is gradually changing. There is a realization that we need to accept death as a natural process.

The process of dying involves a lot of psychological reactions, like:

1. Denial ("Not me").
2. Anger ("Why me?").
3. Bargaining ("Yes me, but").
4. Depression ("Yes, me").
5. Acceptance ("My time is close now, it is all right").

People who know or suspect they are dying may want to talk about it. Often they look for someone to share their fears with. Dying persons need the opportunity to live their final expectations to the fullest. People who are dying remain more or less the same as they were during life. The dying person faces the following tasks:

1. Reviewing life.
2. Coping with physical symptoms in the end stage of life.
3. Making a transition from a known to unknown state and
4. Reacting to separation from loved ones.

Crying and tears are an important aspect of the grief process. The nurse caring for a dying person may have the chance of getting the following negative attitudes or obstacles:

1. Forgetting that a dying person may be feeling lonely, abandoned and afraid of dying.
2. The nurses' unwillingness to share the process of dying and hence minimizing their contacts with the person.
3. Reacting with irritation and hostility to the person's frequent calls.
4. Feeling afraid, uneasy and frustrated in caring for a dying person, the nurse may fail to get the help from her team members.
5. Not allowing the dying person to talk about death and dying.

The above mentioned negative attitudes towards the dying person are what the nurse should learn to avoid. The nurse should assess the physical, psychological and other problems related to a dying person for better terminal care. The nurse should try to support the dying person and his family members. She should try to minimize the physical discomfort, allowing the person and family to do the work of grieving and mourning, allow crying, and expressing of feelings, fears and concerns.

Provide care and comfort with relief from pain. Do not isolate the person. Stay physically close, use touch. Keep activities in room as near normal and constant as possible. Speak in audible tones, not whispers. Be alert to cases when persons need to be alone; leave room for hope. Help a person die with peace of mind by lending support and allowing him to die with dignity.

Chapter

28

Legal Aspects of Psychiatric Nursing

There is an increasing awareness regarding mental health in our population. Along with this, comes an increasing involvement of psychiatry with the law which compels us to focus our attention on this relationship.

The nurse working in a psychiatric set up should realize that law comes into contact with psychiatry at many instances. The law in relation to the mentally ill can only be a reflection of the larger reality relating to the understanding of mental illness and care.

The nurse in a psychiatric hospital should know the following basic forensic psychiatry (legal aspects of psychiatry):

1. Crime and psychiatric disorders.
2. Criminal responsibility.
3. Civil responsibility.
4. Laws relating to psychiatric disorders.
5. Admission procedures of patients in a psychiatric hospital.
6. Nursing responsibility.

Patients who require expert psychiatric opinion in the judiciary are:

1. Those who may harm themselves or society.
2. Those who cannot look after the welfare of their family or property.
3. Those who may turn out to be dangerous if they act upon their abnormal thinking.
4. Also spouses of mentally ill patients may require a psychiatrists evidence in the court of law in the matter of divorce.

There is now an increasing awareness of rights in our democracy, which results in increase in litigation. Civil rights movements and consumer councils are gaining more and more importance in our life time.

Hence, the nurse working with psychiatric patients should be more vigilant. They should have a good understanding of the medicolegal aspects of mental health.

CRIME AND PSYCHIATRIC DISORDERS

The widespread concern over increasing crime rate is very obvious. The role of psychiatry in understanding and modifying this extensive and costly criminal behavior is not clear and is a subject of controversy. Traditionally, criminality has been associated with mental illness, though there is no definite evidence.

Mentally ill people can commit a crime due to the following reasons:

1. Some severely mentally ill persons are more hostile than normal people. If the hostility is directed outside it ends up in crime and violence, especially homicide. If the hostility is directed towards self, it becomes suicide.
2. Psychotic patients may act upon the influence of their delusions and hallucinations. They do not have insight, hence, they may not know what they are doing is right or wrong.
3. Psychotic patients and brain damaged persons become more irritable and at times indulge in violence when they are excited.
4. Alcoholics commit crimes either under the influence of alcoholic excitement or during the withdrawal period.
   Alcohol and drug addicts may indulge in robbery, stealing, etc. to get their drugs.
5. Antisocial personality disorder people are prone to criminal behavior because they are basically loveless and guiltless.
6. Mentally retarded persons because of their poor intelligence and uninhibited behavior, are vulnerable and likely to indulge in criminal activity. At times they are exploited by others to commit a crime.
7. Depressed persons when they are totally hopeless and in despair may kill their family members and then commit suicide.
8. Mentally ill people commit crime also due to the problems arising from stress produced in the family and society.
9. Epileptic persons, due to their confusional state, become irritable, excited and are prone to commit crime.

The following few psychiatric disorders are associated with criminal behavior:

Common

1. Schizophrenia.
2. Delusional disorder.
3. Epilepsy.
4. Mental retardation.
5. Alcohol and drug dependence.
6. Antisocial personality disorder.

Rare

1. Affective disorder (mood disorder).
2. Organic mental disorder.
3. Premenstrual tension syndrome.

Various views have been put forth for the association of crime with psychiatric disorders. One view is that the pattern of crime in psychiatric patients is the same for the general population. Males outnumber females in criminal acts.

CRIMINAL RESPONSIBILITY OF MENTALLY ILL PERSONS

According to Section 84 of the Indian Penal Code "Nothing is an offence which is done by a person, who at the time of doing it, by reason of unsoundness of mind, is incapable of knowing the nature of the act, or that he is doing what is either wrong or contrary to law".

It is under this provision that a mentally ill person is exempted from punishment for an offence. At the time of the act, he is suffering from mental illness hence he is not:

a. Having the capacity to understand his act and
b. Aware that it is against law.

This act is based on the famous McNaughton's rule of England.

Civil Responsibility

In a court of law all persons are considered, to be sane (normal) unless otherwise proved. Psychiatric patients, by virtue of their mental illness, are deprived of certain civil rights.

1. Testamentary capacity: If a person suffers from mental illness at the time of making his will and if he does not have the mental capacity to understand the consequences of the act, his will becomes invalid.
2. Marriage: As per the Hindu Marriage Act, a marriage with a person who is a mentally retarded or a mentally ill at the time of marriage can be declared null and void. The spouse can appeal for judicial separation or divorce.
3. Witness: A mentally ill person is not allowed to be a witness in the court of law.
4. Mentally ill person cannot transfer his property or sell his property to others.
5. A mentally ill person cannot stand for the election and he cannot vote.
6. A mentally ill person cannot enter into a business contract.

LAWS RELATING TO PSYCHIATRY IN INDIA

I. The Indian Lunacy Act, 1912.
II. The Mental Health Act, 1987.
III. The Mental Health Care Act, 2012 Draft.

The Indian Lunacy Act, 1912 has been the governing act for many years in India. Presently, it is in the process of being replaced by the Mental Health Act, 1987.

The Mental Health Act, 1987 is the act that governs the welfare of mentally ill in our country. It controls the procedures of treatment and care of the mentally ill. This act has provisions which take care of the property and other affairs of the mentally ill. It protects the human rights of the mentally ill.

The Mental Health Act has 10 chapters dealing with various matters connected with mentally ill people. This act uses the term mentally ill person which was earlier known as lunatic. The word lunatic asylum is replaced by the word psychiatric hospital. A criminal lunatic is now known as mentally ill prisoner.

Admission Procedures in Psychiatric Hospital

Admission procedures of mentally ill persons in a psychiatric hospital differs from admission of patients with physical diseases in a general hospital.

The reasons are:

1. Some of the persons who suffer from major mental illnesses are not aware that they are mentally ill (lack of insight). Hence, they do not seek medical help and at times even refuse treatment.
   Then, it is the responsibility of the relatives and authorities to give them psychiatric care.
2. By virtue of their illnesses some people are at times dangerous to themselves and to others. Hence, they have to be admitted by the authorities and relatives.
3. A lot of medicolegal problems are associated with the mentally ill. Hence, they should be properly channelized for admission. Care also should be taken that no sane (normal) person is admitted by someone with an ulterior motive.
4. Admissions of mentally ill prisoners (criminals) are done with proper procedure.

In India, admission procedures of mentally ill persons in psychiatric hospitals are governed by the Mental Health Act, 1987. As per the Act, the admission in psychiatric hospitals or nursing home is to be done in one of the following manner:

1. Voluntary admission
   a. On the patient's request, if he is a major.
   b. By the parent or legal guardian if he is a minor.
2. Admission under special circumstances: This is involuntary admission. It is done when the mentally ill person does not or cannot express his willingness for admission. The duration for admission cannot exceed 90 days.
3. Reception order on petition: By a petition from the patient's relatives, followed by certification by two doctors and a reception order from a magistrate.
4. Reception order other than on petition: Admission of a dangerous and wandering person by a reception order from a judicial magistrate or by a commissioner of police.
5. Judicial Inquisition (Enquiry).
6. Admission of mentally ill prisoners (criminal lunatics): Three types of admissions can be made through a reception order. An order under:
   a. The Prisoners Act III, 1900: Mentally ill prisoner who becomes mentally ill during their imprisonment (convicts).
   b. Section 330 of the Criminal Procedure Code: Persons who committed a crime but is not in a position to stand for trial because of his impaired mental functions (under trial prisoners).
   c. Section 335 of the Criminal Procedure Code: Persons who committed a crime due to their mental illness. They are guilty (accepts their crime) but are mentally ill. Hence, they are not given punishment but admitted in a psychiatric hospital for treatment (guilty but insane).

Special Admission Procedures for Military Persons

1. Section 144 of The Air Force Act, 1950.
2. Section 145 of The Army Act, 1950.
3. Section 143 or 144 of The Navy Act, 1957.

DISCHARGE PROCEDURE

For civil patients: A person has to be discharged if he applies for discharge within 24 hours in the case of voluntary admission. A relative or guardian can also apply. The discharge of the civil patients admitted through reception orders has to be made by the visiting committee.

Discharge of mentally ill prisoners (Criminals): Persons admitted under Section 335 CPC can be discharged by the Criminal Committee after a stipulated time and if the person has been showing continued improvement in his mental status. Persons admitted under Section 330 and Act III is to be sent back to prison after improvement.

The responsibility of the nurse in a psychiatric hospital:

1. The nurse should have a good understanding of the law related to psychiatry.
2. She should have a good knowledge of the admission procedure of the mentally ill in a psychiatric hospital.
3. In view of the medicolegal aspects of psychiatric cases, case files are to be kept under safe custody. She should maintain confidentiality about her patient's particulars.
4. She should be watchful and sincere in her duties, not only to give better care of the patient, but also because of the implication" of the civil rights movement and consumer councils.
5. The nurse should get informed consent from patient and/or his relatives before:
   a. Admission on voluntary basis.
   b. Electroconvulsive therapy.
   c. Disulfiram therapy in alcoholism and pentathol analysis (narco analysis).

   These procedures carry some risks, like risk to life, risk of fracture, etc.

   A written consent from the patient (on a specified form provided for the purpose), if he is able to sign, should always be taken. If he is unable to sign, the form must be signed by his guardian or by both, the patient and a close relative.

   Before getting the consent of the patient or his legal guardian, full explanation is necessary with regard to the risks involved in the treatment to be given to the patient.
6. Nurses working in a ward, where mentally ill prisoners are admitted should be very watchful for attempt to escape. These patients may also have suicidal and/or homicidal tendencies. This should be recognized and watched carefully.

MENTAL HEALTH CARE ACT, 2012–DRAFT

Ministry of Health and Family Welfare, Government of India, New Delhi.

Overview and Comments

The government of India, Ministry of Health and Family Welfare has brought out a draft of the Mental Health Care Act 2012 based on the inputs from the five regional consultations and those provided by the professional bodies and other stake holders.

Mental health care in India is gaining a momentum in the recent past. Almost every aspect of life in the modern days is regulated or affected in some way by Law. Most of the civilization in the world has enacted laws to regulate human behavior, so that, the weakest can live freely and enjoy all his human rights. There is a dynamic relationship between the concept of mental illness, the treatment of the mentally ill, and the law.

In the Indian context, many acts are directly or indirectly related to mental health. Currently, the Mental Health Act 1987 (MHA 87) is a major legislation and it has become supposed to be operational in 1994 in all states of the Indian Union, but, only after the Erwadi tragedy in 2004 many states started implementing, as per the order of the Supreme Court. This Act replaces the Indian Lunacy Act, 1912.

Even though, lot of new developments and modifications have been included in the MHA 87, many of the mental health professionals, NGOs, and other stake holders felt there are lot of lacunae and deficiencies in this Act. Hence, in the last 15 years, many organizations including Indian Psychiatric Society consumers started demanding a new Act which can fulfill the aspirations and improve the quality of care of the mentally ill. Based on this, the Government of India, Ministry of Health has taken steps to bring about a new Act, Mental Health Care Act, 2012. (MHCA 2012) and after wide consultations released the draft on December 6, 2012. This draft will take a final shape after suggestions and some more recommendations, which will then be circulated to the Law Ministry and later the Bill will be introduced in both houses of Parliament. The bill should be passed in both the houses and it will be enacted after getting the President of India's approval.

The basic requirements of a new Mental Health Act:

- A comprehensive mental health policy of the government drafted in consultation with professional bodies
- Incorporation of modern concept of psychiatry
- Basic statutory structure of mental health legislation as laid down in the guiding principles and alternative approaches recommended by the WHO
- Apart from the care of the mentally ill and their rights the act should comprise facilities to promote mental health programme
- Should take into account the care of the common (minor) mental disorders
- The new MHA should focus on community psychiatry and rehabilitation programs
- Should coordinate with other agencies/institution to increase human resources in the field of mental health
- Same standard should be prescribed for both government and private psychiatric facilities
- Provisions should be made available for special groups like elderly, destitute women, etc.

- There should be provisions to monitor effective functioning of the central and State Mental Health Authorities.

The draft of the Mental Health Care Act, 2012, consists of 9 chapters and 67 sections. The proposed Act is more comprehensive, specific, and consumer oriented. This Act resembles some of the advanced countries legislations in that sense, that very great importance is given to the rights of persons with mental illness. The Act's concern to give a quality Mental Health Care and to treat the persons with mental illness with humanity and dignity is evidenced by Chapter II, wherein the various rights of persons with mental illness has been detailed. They are:

- Right to access mental health care
- Right to community living
- Right to protection from cruel inhuman and degrading treatment
- Right to equality and nondiscrimination
- Right to information
- Right to confidentiality
- Access to medical records
- Right to personal contacts and communication
- Right to legal aid
- Right to make complaints about deficiencies in provision of services.

In the title description of Mental Health Care Act, 2012, it is described as an Act to provide access to mental health care for persons with mental illness and to protect and promote the rights of persons with mental illness during the delivery of mental health care. Hence, it is understood that the two important objectives of this MHCA 2012 are access to mental health care and protection and promotion of rights of persons with mental illness. Unlike the MHA, the present Act talks about rehabilitation also as a part of the care.

In the Chapter I, where the definitions are prescribed lot of new concepts have been included like caregiver, informed consent, least restrictive alternative or less restrictive option, mental health facility, mental health professional, mental health review commission, and district panel of the mental health review commission have all been included.

The definition of mental illness is more specific and comprehensive compared to MHA 87. This Act defines mental illness as "a disorder of mood, thought, perception, orientation or memory which causes significant distress to a person or impairs a person behavior, judgment, and ability to recognize reality or impairs the person's ability to meet the demands of normal life and includes mental conditions associated with the abuse of alcohol and drugs, but excludes mental retardation."

In section 4 of Chapter I, the concept of competence or competent to make a decision has been very clearly put forth. In section 5, a new concept of advance directive has been specified. Every person has a right to make an advance directive in writing, specifying any or all of the following:

a. The way the person wishes to be cared for and treated for a mental illness and/or
b. The way the person wishes not to be so cared for and treated for a mental illness and/or
c. The individual or individuals, in order of precedence, the person wants appointed as their nominated representative.

The concept of Advance Directive and Nominated Representative are all going in hands with the modern concept of mental health care delivery. There are different terms like relative, caregiver, guardian, and nominated representative have been mentioned. Even though, they seem to be synonyms each one has a different meaning and purpose in this act. The nominated representative has to be appointed by the district panel of the Mental Health Review Commission and he is responsible for all the legal and health care protection of the person with mentally ill. This term has almost replaced the concept of guardian. In minors, below 18 years, the legal guardian need not always be the nominated representative of the child.

The very positive note in using terminology in this new Act is evidenced by using the phrase "Person with mental illness" rather than using the term "Mentally-ill person", in accordance with the WHO guidelines.

In Chapter III, the duties of government in promoting mental health program and creating awareness about mental health problems and to improve the human resources are mentioned.

The Chapter IV deals with Mental Health Review Commission, (MHRC) this mental health review commission would replace the Central Mental Health Authority of MHA 87. The Central Government shall constitute MHRC within three months of the Act coming into force. This will have the jurisdiction all over the country.

The MHRC consists of:

- A President (High Court Judge)—to be appointed by the President of India
- One Member—a psychiatrist with 15 years experience
- One Member—a representative of persons with mental illness or families or caregivers or NGOs.

Members to be appointed by the Central Government.

Section 22 of Chapter IV describes the constitution of district panels of the mental health review commission (District Panel of MHRC). The MHRC shall appoint and function through the District Panels in the districts.

The District Panels functions as per the guidance of MHRC. Each District Panel of the commission shall consist of:

A. Chairperson—a District Judge.
B. Two members—Mental Health Professionals; of which one shall be a psychiatrist and other a mental health professional.
C. Two members from the stake holders—Either the persons with mental illness or caregivers or representatives of NGOs.

The President of the MHRC shall constitute a committee for each state to appoint members of the District Panel. The State Committee consists of

The President or one of the members of the MHRC—he is the Chairperson.

- Chief Justice of the State or his nominee
- Secretary, Ministry of Law of the State Government or his nominee
- Secretary, Ministry of Health of Family Welfare of the State or his nominee
- Secretary, Ministry of Social Welfare of the State or his nominee.

Any person with mental illness whose rights are violated or his nominated representative or an NGO may make an application to the District Panel for redressal.

Section 28 of Chapter IV describes the functions of MHRC and District Panel of the MHRC.

THE FUNCTIONS OF THE MENTAL HEALTH REHABILITATION CENTER

- Appoint and remove members of District Panel
- Guidance to District Panel
- Periodic review of the use of advance directives
- Advise Central Government on matters relating to the promotion and protection of rights of persons with mental illness.

THE FUNCTIONS OF DISTRICT PANELS OF MENTAL HEALTH REHABILITATION CENTER

- To review, alter, modify and advance directive
- To appoint a nominated representative
- To decide applications from persons with mental illness or caregivers
- To decide applications regarding nondisclosure of information
- To decide complaints regarding deficiencies in the care and services
- To visit prison or jails and question the responsible medical officer taking care of mentally ill.

From the draft, it looks as if the MHRC is replacing the existing Central Mental Health Authority, even though, it is not specifically mentioned in the draft.

Chapter V describes about the formation and functions of the State Mental Health Authority (SMHA). The State Government shall constitute the SMHA within three months of the Act coming into force. The SMHA has totally 13 members. They are:

a. Ex Officio members
    1. Secretary, State Department of Health.
    2. Representative of State Department of Health, who is responsible for mental health.
    3. Head of the mental hospital.
b. Other members:
    1. A prominent psychiatrist from the state, who is not in government service.
    2. A psychiatric social worker.
    3. A clinical psychologist.
    4. A mental health nurse.
    5. Two persons representing persons who have or have had mental illness.
    6. Two persons representing caregivers.
    7. Two persons representing NGOs working in the field of mental health.

The term duration for each member is three years.

Section 34 talks about the executive officer of SMHA (EO of SMHA). The Chairperson (Health secretary) shall appoint an EO to the authority. The EO shall be a full-time employee of the authority. He controls and monitors the functioning of SMHA.

The functions of SMHA are almost like what has been detailed in MHA 87.

Chapter VI deals with mental health facilities. The existing term of psychiatric hospital has been removed, instead, the organization or institution taking care of the mentally ill is now known as the mental health facility. The mental health facilities are categorized and minimum standard of care is provided. The mental health facility is defined (as per Chapter I, Section 2 (h)) as "all facilities either wholly or partly, meant for the care of the persons with mental illness, establish or maintained by the government or any other person or organization, where persons with mental illness are admitted or reside at, or kept in, for care, treatment, convalescence, and/or rehabilitation, either temporarily or otherwise; and includes any general hospital or general nursing home established or maintained by the government or any other person or organization; and excludes a family residential place if a person with mental illness resides with his or her own family".

The mental health facility should obtain registration from the State Mental Health Authority. Hence, the SMHA functions as the licensing as well as inspecting authority unlike in MHA 87. After the State Government fix the standards and categories of mental health facilities and officially notified, the Mental Health Facilities should get their permanent registration within a period of six months.

Chapter VII deals with admission, treatment, and discharge.

Following are the different types of admissions as per Mental Health Care Act, 2012.

- Independent (without support) admission and treatment—at the request of the individual himself
- Admission of a Minor—at the request of the nominated representative.
- Admission and treatment of persons with mental illness, with high support needs, in a mental health facility, up to 30 days (Supported admission).

1. Admission and treatment of persons with mental illness with high support needs, in a mental health facility beyond 30 days (Supported admission beyond 30 days).
2. Admission of wandering mentally ill or a person at risk to himself or to others due to mental illness or a person with mental illness, who is ill-treated or neglected.

It is the duty of the police officer to take these mentally ill persons into protection and produce them before the magistrate for authorizing the admission of the person with mental illness in a mental health facility for such period not exceeding 10 days for assessment and planning of the treatment.

Section 59 deals with admission of prisoners with mental illness.

Section 60 deals with admission of person with mental illness for judicial process.

Section 51 deals with prohibited treatments, where it is mentioned that ECT without muscle relaxant and anesthesia, for minors and during emergency treatment should not be given. Sterilization of men and women shall not be performed when such sterilization is intended as a treatment for mental illness and persons with mental illness shall not be chained.

Section 52 gives the consent and the procedure for psychosurgery for persons with mental illness.

Section 53: Deals with guidelines for restraints and seclusions for unmanageable or risky mentally ill persons.

Chapter IX deals with the penalties and miscellaneous provisions.

Section 61: Deals with penalties for establishing and maintaining a mental health facility in contravention of this Act.

Section 63: Deals with special relaxation applicable for the states of North East Council. There is a provision of MHCA 2012 for emergency treatment for a maximum period of 72 hours by any medical practioner to prevent death or irreversible harm to the health of the person or the person inflicting serious harm to himself or to others or the person causing serious damage to the property belonging to him or others.

COMMENTS

Even though, the modern concept of Mental Health Care has been formed as the basis for this Act, it is better for our Nation to have a comprehensive Mental Health Policy to be framed before any Mental Health Legislation or program to be charted out. There are a lot of positive thinking in defining many terms in Mental Health Care including the mental illness. The qualification of psychiatric social worker and the clinical psychologist should be more specified like "the psychiatric social worker means any person holding MA in social work/MSW/M Phil in social work, who have obtained their Masters Degree in Medical and Psychiatric Social Work in a recognized institution".

The term clinical psychologists means after postgraduation, a recognized qualification in clinical psychology in a recognized institution or an institution attached to a hospital. The term "psychiatric hospital" has been replaced by a comprehensive term "Mental Health Facility". The Mental Health Review Commission to monitor the countries Mental Health Care delivery and the district level panel of this commission will facilitate the smooth functioning of the Mental Health Care Delivery. The term "Licence"; instead, the term "Registration" has come in. The term licensing authority and the inspecting authority have gone. The admission procedures have been modified for betterment. The emphasis of the new Act is mainly given for protection of human rights and delivering dignified quality mental health care to the persons suffering from mental illness.

Mental illness should not be viewed as either a "medical" or "legal" conditions alone, but a sociological dimension has to be incorporated. "Exclusive judicial preoccupation with the medical concept of mental illness is not preferable. Each case has to be considered on its own merits. (Justice Venkatachaliah 1988).

Since law is the King of Kings, nothing can be mighter than the law by whose aid; even the unfortunate mentally ill may have the rights to have equal opportunity, rights to have protection of legal rights and rights to have full participation in the affairs of life on par with those who are nondisabled.

THE ROLE OF THE NURSE IN THE LEGAL ASPECTS OF PSYCHIATRY

Professional nursing practice is not determined by simply following patient's rights. Rather, it is an interplay between the patient's rights, the legal role of the nurse and concern for quality psychiatric care:

Three roles:

1. Provider of services.
2. Employee or contractor of services.
3. Private citizen.

Nurses as Provider

- Duty to warn or protect
- Responsible record keeping
- Informed consent
- Substituted consent
- Confidentiality
- Standard nursing care
- Knowledge of legal aspects.

Nurse as an Employee

- This involves the practitioner rights and responsibilities in relation to employers, partners, consultants, and other professional colleagues
- Economic security
- Professional future and
- Peer relationship.

Nurses as a Citizen

The third role of the nurse play is that of a citizen, the role is particularly significant all other roles, rights, responsibilities and privileges are awarded because of the inherent rights of citizenship. Our form of democratic government, grants their rights as inherent.

Civil rights:

- Property rights
- Rights to protection from harm
- Right to a good name
- Right to due process.

Chapter

29

The Role of a Nurse in Mental Health Practice

The nurse, who is taking care of psychiatric patients is expected to work in different areas, as psychiatric nursing does not mean just the care of mental hospital patients. The care of psychiatric patient extends beyond the walls of the hospital to encompass the needs of patients in other set-ups.

The psychiatric nurse has to be familiar with:
1. Mental hospital psychiatry
2. General hospital psychiatry and
3. Community psychiatry.

In giving care to the mentally ill, none of the above can substitute the other. Instead each system should support the other. Some patients are to be kept only in a mental hospital. Many others have to be attended in a general hospital set-up. Psychiatric care can be given effectively at community level also. Nowadays, looking after the mentally ill patients at home is more encouraged, as it is advised in some other physical illness like tuberculosis.

To improve mental health care in our country all the three systems namely, mental hospital psychiatry, general hospital psychiatry and community psychiatry should have a coordinated and integrated health care plan.

THE NURSE IN A PSYCHIATRIC INSTITUTIONAL (MENTAL HOSPITAL) SETTING

The skills required are:
- Basic nursing skills
- Technical nursing skills
- Occupational and recreational skills
- Organizational skills
- Interpersonal skills
- Observational skills
- Skills of communication with patients and coworkers.

In a psychiatric institutional setting, the nurse may be called upon to work in the:

- Outpatient department of the psychiatric hospital
- Day hospital
- Acute emergency ward
- Family care units
- Special clinics like child guidance clinics, deaddiction wards, etc.
- Rehabilitation units.

THE NURSE IN A MENTAL HOSPITAL HAS A ROLE TO PLAY

- The safe custody of patients
- Carrying out various treatment modalities (physical and psychological)
- The administration of the ward
- Carrying out the therapeutic milieu
- Responsibility of health education to patients and their relatives
- Patient centered and research minded responsibilities
- Maintain better adjustment and cordial relationships with professional colleagues
- Playing an active role in promoting mental health services.

THE NURSE IN THE GENERAL HOSPITAL SETTING

There are many types of duty which may Occur in GH:

- The anxieties of the normal patients suffering from any type of illness
- Those with psychosomatic illness or other types of mild emotional disturbance
- Those with obvious but manageable mental illness
- Those with acute psychiatric disturbance
- Those who attempted suicide.

THE NURSE IN COMMUNITY MENTAL HEALTH SERVICES

The nurse's role in this setting can be viewed from different angles:

Health promotion, which includes:

- Participation in health education programs
- Working with special groups, e.g. pregnant women, elderly, adolescents, etc.
- Helping the authorities in changing the attitude towards mental illness
- Activity with the individual, the family or special groups preventive action and case finding
- Ensuring continuity of care
- Participation in studies with regard to community needs
- Participation in rehabilitation programs.

Chapter

30

General Hospital Psychiatry

A nurse undergoing training in psychiatry should understand that there are three components in psychiatry. They are:

- Mental hospital psychiatry
- General hospital psychiatry and
- Community psychiatry.

It was once considered that psychiatry was equivalent to the study of madness and psychiatric training was training in a mental hospital. This concept has become outdated. More and more people suffer from minor psychological problems and they mostly attend a general hospital for treatment.

It is estimated that in India, 15 to 20 percent of people who seek medical help in primary health centers and general hospitals have some sort of psychological problem, but most of them are not aware of it. They think and believe that they have some physical illness and take a variety of treatment for relief, all in vain.

The common mental health problems seen in a general hospital are:

- Anxiety related disorders
- Depressive illness—mostly masked depression
- Stress related and psychosomatic disorders
- Attempted suicide
- Organic mental disorders like delirium and dementia.

General hospital psychiatry is becoming more and more popular because of many reasons. The two important ones being:

1. The absence or reduction in the stigma associated with seek help for psychological problems.
2. The increasing recognition that psychiatric problems often coexist with physical diseases. The strong relationship between mind and body is getting more recognition in the treatment of physical illnesses.

The general hospital psychiatry is also known as consultation-liaison psychiatry. It is an important and integral element of the general hospital set up. Psychological intervention in general hospital settings not only improves psychiatric morbidity and psychosocial adjustments, but also improves the physical disease. This also reduces the total health care cost.

The interaction between psychiatry and physical illness can be classified under the following headings:

ORGANIC MENTAL DISORDERS

Physical illness has direct effect on brain function.

Examples

- Delirium due to liver or renal failure
- Chronic organic mental disorder-dementia
- Postoperative psychosis
- Toxic psychosis—a psychological disturbance following high fever.

MALADAPTIVE PSYCHOLOGICAL REACTIONS TO ILLNESS

- Depression—following detection of cancer, amputation, stroke, myocardial infarction, etc.
- Guilt—fear of being a burden to relatives
- Anxiety—before operation
- Paranoid reaction—for example, if deaf or blind
- Anger
- Denial—not willing to accept reality
- Preoccupation with illness
- Prolongation of sick role—less responsibility, more attention.

PSYCHOSOMATIC DISORDERS

Multiple causes: Psychobiosocial causes, e.g· stress in a vulnerable person producing or precipitating a physical disease like heart attack, asthma, peptic ulcer, etc.

PSYCHIATRIC CONDITIONS PRESENTING WITH PHYSICAL COMPLAINTS

- Somatic anxiety symptoms (physical symptoms) due to autonomic hyperactivity, e.g. palpitation, tremor, etc.
- Conversion disorder "A psychological or emotional conflict is converted into a physical disorder, e.g. hysterical fit". An attention seeking behavior
- Depression leading to facial pain, hypochondriacal disorders having incurable diseases
- Somatization disorder—physical symptom without any organic basis due to a psychological disturbance, e.g. noncardiac chest pain

- Monosymptomic hypochandrical delusion, e.g. delusion of infestation
- Hospital addiction syndrome (Munchausen's syndrome)
- Alcoholism leading to liver disease.

PHYSICAL CONDITIONS PRESENTING WITH PSYCHIATRIC COMPLAINTS

- Depressive disorder precipitated by cancer
- Anxiety in hyperthyroidism
- Post-viral depression.

MEDICAL DRUGS LEADING TO PSYCHIATRIC COMPLICATIONS

- Antihypertensive drugs leading to depression
- Corticosteroids leading to depression or euphoria
- Antileprosy drug (dapsone) and anti-TB drug (INH) producing psychosis.

PSYCHIATRIC DRUGS LEADING TO MEDICAL COMPLICATIONS

- Over dose of antipsychotic or antidepressive drugs
- Chlorpromazine, inducing jaundice
- Tricycle antidepressants inducing arryhthmias.

As the field of medicine becomes increasingly complex, areas of specialization naturally arise. In a general hospital set up, the role of mental health professional is very much appreciated.

Psychological intervention will facilitate symptom removal and speedy recovery in many medical sub-specialities. The following are the important medical specialities where a mental health professional can be a part of the team in the management.

1. Intensive medical care unit.
2. Intensive coronary care unit.
3. Burns ward.
4. Dialysis units.
5. Cancer wards.
6. Geriatiric unit.
7. Obstetric and gynecology unit especially during postpartum care.
8. Postoperative wards.
9. Cardiothoracic and organ transplantation units.
10. Rehabilitation units.
11. Crisis intervention/suicide prevention clinics.
12. Gastroenterology units.

Psychiatry in the general hospital involves a lot of activities that will improve health care system. The nurses working in the general hospital set-up should understand the following basics:

1. Many physical illnesses have underlying psychological basis.
2. Nursing a physical illness with drugs and other procedure alone may not be sufficient. It requires a psychological approach. When treating a physically ill person, sympathy, care and comfort should be provided to him. Not alone his physical problem, but his emotional problems should be understood and taken care off as well.
3. The nurse should understand that there are three factors influencing any physical illness:
   a. The patient.
   b. The illness.
   c. The social environment.

   Hence, when nursing care is given, there should be a holistic approach.
4. Even when taking care of a physical illness in a general hospital, the nurse should be in a position to give supportive psychotherapy. Not only to the patient, but also to the caregivers. The relatives should also receive psychological comfort and care.

Chapter

31

Stress and Stress Related Disorders (Lifestyle Disorders)

WHAT IS STRESS?

- Stress is a dominant strain in the fabric of today's life
- But what is stress?
- "Stress occurs when people face events that they perceive as endangering their physical and psychological well being"
- These events are known as stressors; and the reaction to them as stress response
- Stress may be minor or major (severe); Short lived or protracted.

DEFINITION

- Stress is a pattern of disruptive physiological and psychological reactions to events that threaten a person's ability to cope
- "A nonspecific response by an organism to demands made on it"
- A certain amount of stress is an in evitable part of life. "Complete freedom from stress is death" (Selye, 1974)
- Stress is something which leads to strain. Stress denotes the psychological side and strain indicates physical side of the same problems.

TYPES OF STRESS

Normal activity causes stress. Stress cannot be avoided, for to be free from stress is to be dead.

Two kinds of stress are there:

1. Eustress—Healing and pleasant
2. Distress—Disease producing and unpleasant.

ACTUALLY WHAT DOES STRESS MEAN IN PRACTICE

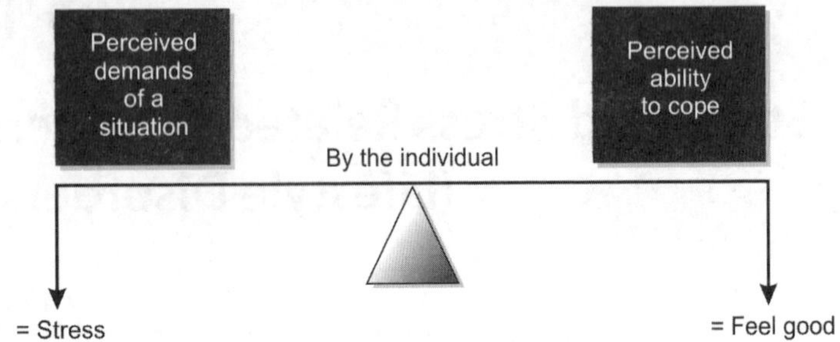

FIGHT OR FLIGHT RESPONSE

Arousal response via hypothalamus to pituitary

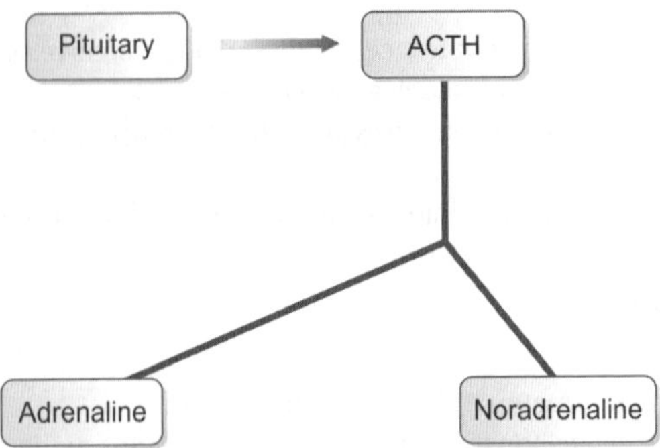

This speeds up of body metabolism and increase autonomic nervous system activity which leads on to fight or flight response.

WHERE STRESS GENERATES FROM?

a. Stress at home:
   1. Marital disharmony, separation or divorce.
   2. Financial difficulties.
   3. Child birth.
   4. Problems in children.
   5. Problems with in laws or parents.
   6. Alcoholism and domestic violence.
b. Work related stress.
c. Social stressors.

STAGES OF STRESS REACTION

- Stage of alarm reaction
- Stage of resistance
- Stage of exhaustion.

LIFE EVENTS AND STRESS

- Performance (in work, family, sex, etc.)
- Bereavement (actual loss of a person or part of one's body)
- Threat (to one's self-esteem, job, security, etc.)
- Physical (disease, malfunctioning, etc.)
- Frustration due to inability to achieve one's desired goal
- Boredom (due to lack of adequate stimulation).

ENVIRONMENTAL CONDITIONS AND LIFESTYLE HABITS RELATED TO STRESS

Environmental factors like high pollution stressful jobs, repeated X-ray exposure, radioactive drugs, and toxic chemical irritants can induce stress in a vulnerable person.

Some of the lifestyle habits like excessive coffee, tea, smoking, alcohol, high fat/sugar diet, hectic lifestyle are some of the factors which may cause stress.

STRESS–INTERACTION MODEL

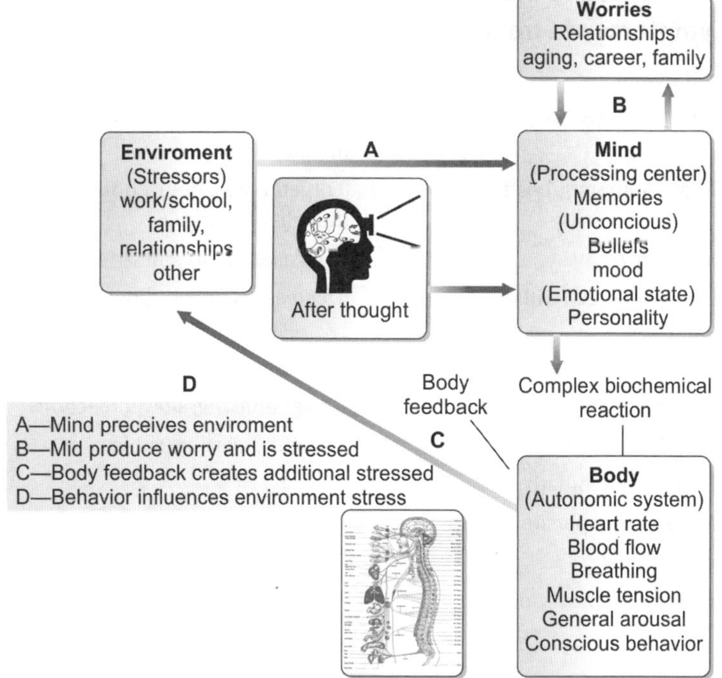

Type A Personality

Persons who are extremely competitive and achievement oriented and consider to be too much ambitious, workaholic are consider to be having type A personality. They are more prone to develop coronary artery diseases.

Physical Signs and Symptoms of Stress

Increased Heart rate	Gastrointestinal problems
Elevated blood pressure	Restlessness, hyperactivity
Tightness of chest	Vague somatic complaints
Breathing difficulty	Backache
Headaches, migraine	Frequent or prolonged colds or flu
	Bruxism, clenching
Fatigue, exhaustion	Urinary frequency
Insomnia	Weight gain or weight loss

Emotional and Mental Signs and Symptoms of Stress

Emotional	*Intellectual*
Irritability, overreaction	Negative attitude, cynical, job dissatisfaction.
Angry outbursts, hostility	Forgetfulness, preoccupation thought blocking
Jealousy	Increased fantasy life
Lack of interest, withdrawn, apathetic	Decreased concentration
Crying tendencies	Inattention to detail
Blaming others, suspicious attitude	Slower thinking, slower reactions
Self-depreciating	Difficulty learning subjects
Diminished initiative	
Reduction of personal involvement with others	
Depression, worrying	

Various Stress-Related Diseases and Conditions (Lifestyle Disorders)

System affected	Resulting condition
Cardiovascular system	Coronary artery disease, Hypertension, Stroke, rhythm disturbances of the heart
Muscular system contraction backache	Tension headaches, muscle
Locomotor system	Rheumatoid arthritis
Respiratory and allergic disorders	Asthma, Hay fever
Immunological disorders	Lowered resistance, autoimmune diseases
Gastrointestinal disturbances	Peptic ulcer, Irritable bowel syndrome Diarrhoea, Ulcerative colitis
Genitourinary disturbances	Diuresis, impotence, frigidity
Dermatological diseases	Eczema, neurodermatitis, acne
Other problems	Fatigue and lethargy

COPING SKILLS

- Problem focused coping
- Emotion focused coping
  - Behavioral strategies
  - Cognitive strategies
  - Distraction strategies
  - Negative avoidant strategies
  - Defense mechanism as emotion focused coping

  (Anxiety preventing mechanism with an element of self-deception. Repression, rationalization, reaction formation, projection, denial, displacement, intellectualization).

THE HOLISTIC APPROACH TO THE CONTROL OF STRESS

- Techniques to minimize the frequency of the stress response
- Techniques to minimize the intensity of the stress response and reduce emotional reactivity
- Techniques to utilize stress and promote body consciousness.

MANAGING STRESS

- Behavioral techniques
  - Bio-feedback training
  - Relaxation training
  - Aerobic exercises
- Cognitive techniques
  - Cognitive behavior therapy
- Modifying type A behavior.

RELAXATION TECHNIQUES

- Autogenic
- Self hypnosis
- Yoga
- Meditation.

CORRECTION OF THINKING MISTAKES

- Tunnel vision
- Black and white thinking
- Over-generalization
- Faulty assumptions.

TECHNIQUES TO MINIMIZE THE FREQUENCY OF THE STRESS RESPONSE

- Social engineering
- Personality engineering.

Such program has to be

- Individualized
- Based upon personal preferences and practices
- Multidimensional and
- Flexible.

SOCIAL ENGINEERING STRATEGIES

1. Establish routine when possible.
2. Use time-blocking techniques (for important works).
3. Establish a "mental health day".
4. Remember that a vacation does not always mean relaxation.
5. If possible avoid or minimize other changes during periods of massive changes.

STRESS CAN AFFECT HEALTH

1. Excessive stress is harmful to health. It is one of the most debilitating factors in medical and social problems today.
2. 50% of general medical patients are suffering from stress related problems like headache, high BP muscle tension, perspiration, palpitation, heart problems, diarrhea, diabetes, etc.
3. Stress can also produce mental health problems.
4. Reduce your stress through proper stress management and live a happy, healthy life.

Chapter

32

Disaster and Mental Health Nursing

WHO defines "Disaster" as "Any occurrence that causes damage, economic destruction, loss of human life and detoriation in health services on a scale sufficient to warrant an extraordinary response from outside the affected community or area". Definitions and categorization of disasters vary according to geo-sectors, the geographical and social settings in which they are located.

Disasters can be classified into

Natural
- a. Acute onset—earthquake, cyclones, tsunami, floods, etc.
- b. Chronic onset—Draught, famine, deforestation, and chronic exposure to toxic substances.

Human-Made—For example, war, nuclear explosion, industrial accidents, and other vehicular accidents.

HEALTH CONSEQUENCES OF DISASTERS

1. Disasters may cause an unexpected number of deaths, injuries, or Illness in the affected community.
2. They may destroy health infrastructures such as hospitals.
3. Some disasters may have adverse effects on the environment and the population, increasing the potential risk for communicable diseases.
4. Disasters may affect the psychological and social behavior of the stricken community.
5. Some disasters may cause a shortage of food with severe nutritional consequences.
6. Disasters may cause large, spontaneous or organized population movements.

MAJOR DISASTERS HAPPENED IN INDIA

1. Bhopal gas tragedy.
2. Gujarat earth quake.
3. Orissa greater cyclone.
4. Tsunami in South India.
5. Earth quake in Kashmir.

ROLE OF NURSES IN PROVIDING OUTREACH HEALTH SERVICES DURING EMERGENCIES

Disasters usually have a devastating impact on peoples' lives. In addition, health systems often collapse and access to primary health care services becomes either limited or completely unavailable. In such situations, a nurse can fulfill the following responsibilities:

- Being the first contact of the community with a health care provider
- Educate the community on vital health issues
- Serve as a vital link between the community and the health system
- Provider of "holistic" care, in terms of addressing psychosocial and environmental health issues in addition to providing selected primary health care services and appropriate referral.

EMOTIONAL IMPACT OF DISASTERS

Psychological disturbances following disaster:

- Acute stress reaction
- Grief reaction
- Depression
- Post-traumatic stress disorder. (PTSD) and other anxiety disorders
- Exacerbation of substance sue disorder (especially alcohol abuse).

POST-TRAUMATIC STRESS DISORDER

Along with relief, rehabilitation and the care of the physical health and injuries, mental health issues are also of utmost importance and that need to be addressed.

Any disaster affects people emotionally. The change it brings in life seems unbearable and people often feel helpless, hopeless, and frustrated in the aftermath of a disaster. Often they seem unable to cope with the consequences of the loss they have experienced. They may have repeated thoughts about the events which sort of drains them of energy, this is specially true when they have experienced some violence say in a riot or war, it may leave them feeling very angry and irritable. Survivors may develop revengeful feelings.

Fear is another reaction seen among survivors of disaster. There is fear for its recurrence and this can lead to continued feelings of anxiety, sleeplessness and inability to find strength to regain confidence to lead a normal life.

After an earthquake people continued sleeping outdoors for many days on end and some did not go to the upper stories of their homes.

After communal riots any loud sound would disturb people and they would think it was a bomb, smoke would bring about anxiety and many parents have stopped their children from playing outside after dark.

Grief and depression are commonly seen among survivors of a disaster specially if they have lost family members or friends or at times even animals and material loss. Sometimes, these emotions can develop into suicidal feelings too. Many people want to stay by themselves lose interest in life. Others may take up some substance abuse like alcohol or drugs.

The therapeutic stages include:

- Enduring: anxiety preservation and survival
- Suffering: pain, grieving, insecurity, and loss of the past
- Acceptance: Reality testing, preparedness, and reckoning of the future
- Reconciling: Evaluation of self and resources, recuperating
- Recovery: Rebuilding life, maximizing options. Settle new goals, healing Normalizing stability, routines, building relationships and community.

THE PSYCHOLOGICAL RESPONSE TO A DISASTER DEPENDS ON THREE MAIN FACTORS

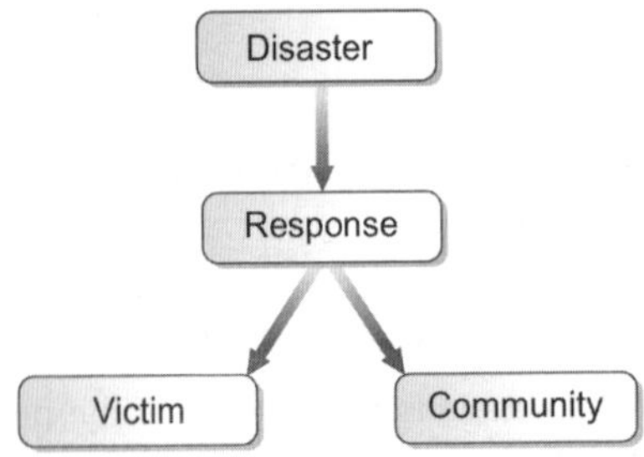

The disaster	The community	The victims
Occurrence	Level of preparedness	Age
Magnitude	Social support	Level of education/ exposure
Suddenness	Leadership	Marital status
Type	Past experience	physical health
		Personality
		Coping skills
		Losses
		Social support

The psychological reactions that people experience as a result of the disaster may be either adaptive or maladaptive. Adaptive responses allow individuals to overcome the difficulties caused by the disaster for instance obtaining information or developing effective survival skills.

Maladaptive reaction include denial, ineffective actions, etc. maladaptive reactions can be prevented from occurring and if they do occur then they can be treated.

Rehabilitation phase is when the population returns to their lives as closely as possible to the pre-disaster situation. Action is taken during this period to re-establish normal activity as much as possible. This begins after the disaster impact and lasts for several hours to four weeks.

Reconstruction phase is the longer period when the population rebuilds personal skills, social support, and leadership. This overlaps with the rebuilding phase.

EMOTIONAL PROBLEM OF CHILDREN

Disasters like the tsunami cause many kinds of psychological and physical disturbances in children. They become helpless, confused not knowing what to do nor help themselves like adults to the extent possible to overcome the impact of tsunami. Disaster cause varied nature of emotional and adjustment problems. These children usually have lost their homes, schools, and some have lost their kith and kin like parents, siblings and pet animals and are deprived of food, clothing and love and affection of their parents and others. They are exposed to unbearable environmental conditions.

BEHAVIOR PROBLEMS

- Repeatedly talking about the disaster
- Behavior like bedwetting, thumb sucking
- Refusal of food
- Sleep problems
- Some appear talking to self or others
- Some children may show problems relating to stealing, lying and disobedient
- Verbal and physical aggression in some
- Poor school work, smoking and other behaviors
- Withdrawal behaviors
- Refusal to attend school.

HOW CAN NURSES HELP THESE CHILDREN

Nurses can play a vital role in meeting the psychosocial needs of these children. The goals of nurses include monitoring the stress levels and trying to reduce them, advocating to prevent serious short- and long-term emotional trauma and rehabilitate the children as much as possible.

You can do the following:

1. Demonstrate consistency in your response to the children and ensure consistency among all the staff members.

2. Convey feeling of empathy to children and family members.
3. Workout a daily schedule for each group of children for performing daily activities.
4. Help the child to be with familiar people like parents, siblings and neighbors.
5. Reassure security to the child by touching, padding, sitting with him.
6. Facilitating the routine environment to the children by encouraging them to play, attend school and develop relationship with teachers, peer groups, eat, sleep and play, etc.
7. Encourage the child to talk about his/her feelings, openly discuss his/her thoughts and feelings related to experience of tsunami.
8. Identity their kith and kin and make arrangements to stay with them.
9. Involve children in play activities, peer group activities.
10. Provide them the reading materials, encourage them in art and drawing activities, singing and modeling, etc.
11. Offer them frequent exercise and motor activities.
12. Allow them to make opportunities to make choices.
13. Discuss with them the abstractions such as moral of stories or movies.
14. Actively listen to and encourage the expression of needs and goals.

BEHAVIOR AND EMOTIONAL PROBLEMS OF ADOLESCENCE

The following are some of the behavioral and emotional problems of adolescents:

1. Helplessness, hopelessness and worthlessness.
2. Palpitation and increased heart beat.
3. Poor or decreased appetite.
4. Smoking.
5. Alcohol consumption.
6. Depression and suicidal ideation.
7. Tension, anxiety, and panic attacks.
8. Disturbance in inner turmoil, self-depreciation and guilt.
9. Rebellious behavior.
10. School refusal and under achievement in school.
11. Withdrawal from social contacts.
12. Verbal and physical aggression.

EMOTIONAL AND BEHAVIOR PROBLEMS OF ADULTS

The following are some of the emotional and behavior problems:

1. Denial.
2. Shock.
3. Tension and anxiety.
4. Panic reactions.
5. Despair.

6. Guilt or blame.
7. Overt alertness.
8. Avoidance.
9. Somatic problems.
10. Excessive use of alcohol and smoking.
11. Withdrawal and isolation.
12. Sadness and crying.

ELDERLY INDIVIDUALS

Elderly disasters survivors experience different kinds of psychosocial problems. They might have lost their immovable and movable materials, which are of great value to them.

WHAT A NURSE CAN DO?

a. As a nurse, analyze the situation of the victim and as a first step, give importance to physical needs of the individual.
   - If he has problem in housing, arrange for same by coordinating with concerned authority.
   - Take care of the basic needs like food, safe drinking water, etc.
   - Offer first aid measures for injured individuals as mentioned in previous chapter on care of injury.
b. Listening: Given importance to what he/she wants to talk. Encourage to express freely on their experience on the impact of tsunami
   - During listening, give importance to the content of talk/feeling
   - Maintain eye to eye contact with survivor when he/she is talking
   - Responds positively during listening – expressing that you understand what they are saying by nodding head, conveying your acceptance that you are following their feelings
   - Do not interrupt them while talking, give time to express their feelings completely
   - Give leading questions of necessary so that to make them elaborate on a particular issue which needs clarification.
c. Allow Ventilation:
   - Most of the individuals who experienced after effect of disaster will have strong emotional feelings which are suppressed due to lack of appropriate opportunity for them to express their feelings
   - These suppressed emotional feeling needs to be released otherwise the pressure keeps building inside and the person may break down one day
   - Hence, it is important for nurses to help these individuals to express their feelings that they have experienced and share the emotions.

This will help them to release their pent-up emotions and thus get relieved

- Sit with them, actively listen to them, they may express about the grief of loss caused to them, it helps you to understand the problems and facilitate you to recognize his or her routines in life
- Empathy is understanding the experience of another person and perceiving what kind of problem the other person is undergoing
  - As a nurse you should
  - Try to be in the person's place or situation, so that you will be able to understand and experience the pain and agony of tsunami affected individuals
  - Try to realize what the survivors (of tsunami) emotional feeling
  - Help in sharing his/her problems and you can empathize with them and can facilitate the emotional support to him/her

d. Externalize the Interest:
- This means diverting the attention and preoccupation of survivors to other areas
- Help them to involve in other activities which he/she is interested. For example, involve them in helping others, organizing some sort of cleaning activities, helping the disabled children, etc. This will divert their mind and they will that they are productive and doing useful activities.

OTHER POSSIBLE INTERVENTIONS

Relaxation and Recreation

- Once you engage them in daily routine, it is important to provide for them some sort of relaxation and recreation
- Involve them in recreational activities like group singing, bhajans, listening to radio, playing games, reading books, etc., which will help them in relief and relaxation so that they feel energetic not lethargic.

Offering Support

- Each and every survivors feel lonely, deserted, isolated having met with after effects of tsunami
- Help them to by providing emotional and physical supports
- Get the support of neighbors, friends, and other voluntary workers
- Utilize the local resources and facilities physical and emotional support to them.

Encourage religious and spiritual activities:
Everyone believes in God, or spiritual powers. It is important for you to encourage them in spiritual activities.

- Organize spiritual discourses by involving religious leaders from Hindu, Muslim, Christian communities
- Facilitate prayer meetings regularly in the shelters, or in colonies meant for them
- Organize bhajans and religious discourses in groups
- Involving in spiritual activities enhances their process of recovery
- Encourage positive lifestyles.

IMMEDIATE PSYCHOSOCIAL CARE

- Remove the panic stricken from the main group and place them with someone who can be nurturing to them
- Listen with concerns to the personal experiences of each survivor whenever possible
- Meet the immediate basic needs like food, safety drinking water, privacy, etc.
- Encourage catharsis of feeling of despair, anxiety loss and grief related issues
- Encourage religious activities
- Facilitate contacts with other family members, community members, leaders, volunteers, etc.
- Provide information about social financial, health and other resources
- Assign them the small supervised tasks in order to help them to occupy their body and mind.

CRISIS REDUCTION COUNSELING

This involves helping each individual identify things they can do to lessen his/her impact caused by disaster such as planning for their future life, procuring of food, clothing, shelter needs for the next day, week, or month.

CRISIS INTERVENTION

This involves offering immediate help or counseling to disaster survivors to help them to resolve their problem as much as possible and to cope with the present problems or emotional disturbances.

This also involves helping them in resuming a state of functioning positively.

EDUCATION

Educate them frequently regarding the typical responses that are expressed following the tsunami. Educate the survivors that the reactions expressed by them are normal reactions to an abnormal situation.

Give information that most people experience and master these reactions, so that the path to recovery and rehabilitation becomes much easier.

The nurses can help these survivors by helping the affected people to recognize and understand the tsunami experiences and the change that they are experiencing in their body and mind. Nurses can also give practical support to rebuild their sheltered lives in the areas of housing, livelihood, health and community life. Your willingness and commitment for this cause is very much essential and needed.

PSYCHOLOGICAL FIRST AID

Psychological first aid (PFA) is one of the specific interventions recommended in a disaster situation. PFA is a "humane", supportive response to a fellow human being, who is suffering and may need support. " It is a set of principles to guide community members dealing with others who have been through events that may be traumatic. PFA involves the following themes:

- Providing practical care and support in a way that does not intrude
- Assessing needs and concerns
- Helping people to address basic needs (for example, food and water, information)
- Listening to people, but not pressuring them to talk
- Comforting people and helping them to feel calm
- Helping people connect to information, services and social supports
- Protecting people from further harm.

PSYCHOLOGICAL DEBRIEFING

Psychological debriefing is promoting ventilation by asking a person to briefly but systematically recount his or her perceptions, thoughts, and emotional reactions during a recent stressful event. The Sphere Project and IASC have reviewed the literature on the effectiveness of psychological first aid and psychological debriefing and found that debriefing may be retraumatizing and worse than no intervention and therefore is not recommended.

Chapter

33

Stigma and Mental Illnesses

INTRODUCTION

Stigma is considered a symbol of disgrace or infamy or reproach attributed to someone.

The Oxford English Dictionary (2005) says "A mark of disgrace or infamy", a sign of severe censure or condemnation; regarded as Impressed on a person or thing; a brand". By Stigma, individuals are devalued, shunned, or otherwise "lessened in their life chances".

Stigma is a broad and multidimensional concept. One of the definitions states: "We are discussing the entire field of people who are regarded negatively, some for having violated....rules, others just for being the sort of people they are or having traits that are not highly valued". (Birenbaum and Sagarin 1976).

To Katz (1979) "Stigma encompasses a perception of a negative characteristic and a global devaluation of the possessor of the characteristic. Issues of isolation and rejection and subsequent prejudice and discrimination, arise from the fact we often try to avoid interaction with individuals whose bodily and psychological characteristics deviate from our own group norms. Stigma is generally ineradicable and irreversible and is implied in terms like "ex-mental" patients or "ex-convicts". In fact, stigma may follow us through a life cycle. (Ainly, et al. 1986). They are denied "Access to the humanizing benefit of free and unfettered social intercourse," (Alonzo and Reynolds, 1995).

Work on stigma refers to the causes, forms and effects of stigma in contemporary society. Stigma, Goffman says is best explained as 'deviation from prevalent or valued 'norms'. Goffman's hypothesis implies that the stigmatized are passive and are victimized. The changes in the 'consciousness' or the psyche of the stigmatized are 'far reaching', a lower self-esteem, the persistent preoccupation with the deficit, a strong current of anger and acquisition of new, total and undesirable identity'. (Murphy,). The features of stigma are to be found both in the individuals and their social milieu. The former is the 'felt' stigma and the latter 'enacted' stigma.

STIGMA AND MENTAL DISORDERS

Stigmatization of people with mental disorders has persisted throughout history. It is manifested by bias, distrust, stereotyping, fear, embarrassment, anger, and/or avoidance or working with, renting to, or employing people with mental disorders, especially severe disorders such as schizophrenia. It reduces patient's access to resources and opportunities (e.g. housing, jobs) and leads to low self-esteem, isolation, and hopelessness. It deters the public from seeking and wanting to pay for care. In its most overt and conspicuous form, stigma results in outright discrimination and abuse. More tragically, it deprives people of their dignity in society.

Stigma against mental illness is probably as old as the civilization itself. There are references to discrimination on the basis of mental illness in almost all the ancient books of law. In the well known Indian Classic "Laws of Manu," there are references to insane persons (UNMATTA) in the chapters related to marriage inheritance, feast after death, rules regarding contract and appearance as a witness, etc.

"We are fortunate enough if we are born without any stigmatizing disabilities like blindness, stunted growth, deafness and mentally deranged" says Avvaiyar, the Tamil Poet, 2000 years back.

The stigma is at its worst against the mentally ill. The dehumanizing stance towards the mentally ill has been summed up thus: "The mentally ill individual appears as a collection of symptoms, not as a person; or if he appears as a person, he looks as if he or she belongs to a special species to be differentiated from the rest of humanity, and put into the insane asylum—the psychiatric hospital as a zoological garden with many differentiated species". (ARIETI, 1950). The stigma against the mentally ill is therefore obvious. Though the mental institutions have improved architecturally, administratively and therapeutically, and though a number of them are dismantling, the change is not appreciable enough in many. The thick cloud of stigma engulfs psychiatric disorders especially of the severe varieties of "psychoses". For example, Schizophrenia.

As is well known, ignorance or lack of proper knowledge is the root cause of all stigma. People assume that everyone who has received a particular diagnosis or treatment is identical. In fact, individuals with the same diagnosis or receiving same treatment may manifest different kinds of symptoms. Even when the symptoms are the same, they may vary widely in their severity.

Perhaps one of the strongest prejudice against mental illness is the fear of violence by mentally ill.

Mental disorders and violence are closely linked with public mind. A combination of factors promotes this perception: sensationalized reporting—by the media whenever a violent act is committed by a former mental patient, popular misuse of psychiatric terms (such as "psycho or psychopathic") and exploitation of stock formulas and narrow stereotypes by the assumption of danger.

One of the problems with the antipsychotic drugs has been the powerful side effects. More than the symptoms of schizophrenia, many times the patients were socially isolated due to the marked extrapyramidal symptoms like stooping gait, masked facies, poverty of movements, etc., due to their medication in the past. Fortunately, in this decade, we are on the threshold of a psychotherapeutic revolution with the arrival of atypical antipsychotic drugs like clozapine, risperidone, olanzapine, etc., which do not produce that serious extrapyramidal symptoms. Even though, they produce different side effects, (metabolic) profile. This has given us an opportunity to fight the stigma against mental illness.

STIGMA AND SEEKING HELP FOR MENTAL DISORDERS

Nearly two-thirds of all people with diagnosable mental disorders do not seek treatment. Stigma surrounding the receipt of mental health treatment is among the many barriers that discourage people from seeking treatment. Concern about stigma appears to be heightened in rural areas in relation to larger towns or cities.

One of the chief obstacles to the successful treatment of schizophrenia and to improving the quality of life of people who suffer from the disorder is the stigma often associated with it. Stigma can lead to severe discrimination, to a delay in seeking and obtaining help and to the exacerbation of the disorder.

Much stigma stems from widespread public misconceptions. A significant proportion of professionals and the general public, as well as decision-makers believes that nobody recovers from schizophrenia and that its symptoms cannot be controlled and the people with the disorder are usually violent, dangerous, lazy, unreliable and unable to work.

The stigma associated with mental illness is strong but generally increases the more an individual's behavior differs from that of the norm. Although, recent advances in psychiatry have increased the understanding of psychiatric disorders, many people with chronic or severe psychiatric disorders may be unaware that effective treatment is available.

Ignorance and stigma may prevent mentally ill persons or their families from seeking appropriate help. Help seeking behavior is determined to a large extent by community attitudes and beliefs about the illness. Blame for the illness may sometimes be placed on the patient or their families. Mental health problems are also sometimes understood as character weakness than real illness that requires proper health care—the mentally ill are thought to be dangerous and likely to have a criminal record. In addition to the obvious distress of seeing a loved one disabled by the consequences of a mental disorder, family members are also exposed to further stigma and discrimination. Medical insurances seem unwilling to pay for the treatment of mental illness, thus creating more financial burden to individuals who are mentally ill and their families.

SUMMARY OF THE STUDY OF STIGMA OF MENTAL ILLNESS IN THIRD WORLD COUNTRIES—AN APPRAISAL

The understanding of stigma of mental disorders in the third world comes from three sources.

A. From studies of the differences in the course and outcome of mental disorders.
B. From the attitude studies.
C. From specific studies of the experience of stigma by patients and their families. It is only in the recent times that the specific studies of stigma has been undertaken in countries like Egypt, Ethiopia, and India.

1. There is sufficient evidence to point out that lack of education is associated with greater stigma and discrimination.
2. Similarly, people in the urban areas experience stigma more than those living in rural areas.
3. Women as a group, both as patients and carers, experience more stigma. Lack of services promotes stigma and discrimination.
4. One important stigma seen to a larger extent in the third world is in relation to the concept of hereditary causation. This is most manifested in the problems of getting married. There is greater degree of stigma associated with socially undesirable behaviors and symptoms, and less with internalizing symptoms. Psychological symptoms carry more stigma than somatic symptoms.

One important obstacle that patients with mental disorders in all regions of the world experience to get access to care is stigma related to their illness. The many sources of stigma are disseminated in different levels throughout communities and professional services. The origin of the term stigma and the historical roots of psychiatry as a medical specialty and of the current concept of mental disorders are important to understand why this phenomenon is so widespread worldwide. Stigma is related to other important phenomena such as stereotype, prejudice, discrimination and social distance and has multiple faces that need to be identified in order to succeed when fighting against stigma.

THE NEEDS OF PEOPLE WITH MENTAL DISORDERS

1. Medical needs.
2. Family needs.
3. Community needs—Avoidance of stigma and discrimination.
4. Rehabilitation needs.

World Health Organization (WHO) emphasized the avoidance of stigma and discrimination as some of the essential needs of people with mental illness.

Stigma is one of the important psychosocial consequences of psychiatric illness. Recently, there has been an increasing focus on stigma related to these illnesses. There is a challenging aspect of psychiatry especially affecting the care of the patients as well as their carers.

Some of the features are: Deinstitutionalization, community care, family courts, advocacy of the rights of the mentally ill—the right for health, consent for treatment, freedom for work, etc. stigma is deeply rooted in society and it is not easy to eradicate it. Adding to these societal attitudes is professional apathy and indifference which only augment the difficulty. Stigma raises the threshold for professional help-seeking and prevents or delays diagnosis and treatment.

WHY STIGMA?

Stigma has many reasons. Some are as follows:

1. Firstly: Mentally ill persons engender a fear in others; a fear that they are dangerous, assaultive and turn violent. To dispel these fears are recent reports indicating that violence is uncommon among the mentally ill hardly exceeding the frequency observed in general population. Earlier, violence was believed to be always associated with mental illness. Violence is generally associated with illness like paranoid schizophrenia and acute affective illness like mania. It is also known that violence is observed in those mentally ill with comorbidity like substance abuse.
2. Secondly: Mental diseases until recently (and even now to some extent) were assumed to be incurable, lasting for life. This means a life-long commitment on the part of carers with the associated consequences.
3. Thirdly: The most distressing feature is the hereditary nature of some of these disorders. The fear of mental illness grips those who would have seen their parents being treated for mental illness years ago that stigma comes into play when certificates of mental illness are issued to patients who become worried whether this would disqualify them for the job.

A stigma towards the mentally afflicted, also affect those closely associated with them and those who treat them is widespread. This is rather strange that it should be so in the era of molecular biology. Discrimination persists especially in selection for jobs, seeking marital alliances, inheritance, role of witnesses in the court of law and in matters of divorce.

MANIFESTATIONS OF STIGMA

- The stigma manifests in many ways and situations. Patient and relatives request to avoid their name and address since the illness may become known to others who might handle the letters
- Some patients do not like their names to be written at the top of psychiatrist's prescription
- While taking an appointment for psychiatric consultation, the name of the person is not furnished
- For patients to seek treatment outside their place of residence to avoid being noticed by local people as frequenting local psychiatrist
- Many a time, psychiatrist finds himself in embarrassing situation while attending the wedding receptions of his patients or other members of his family. The hosts feel uncomfortable by the presence of psychiatrist "How do these people know this doctor? Any one not well in the family?" Such whispers are too common. Hence, it is better that psychiatrist avoid such embarrassments
- Families with mentally ill patients labor under the burden of stigma. Their social activities and interaction with other family members becomes constricted. Many cope with such situations by concealing the fact of mental illness
- The most difficult task the parents face is getting their daughter or a son married. Stigma surfaces more intensely in the context of proposed marital alliances. The fact of mental illness is "suppressed" prior to marriage. However, later such marriages prove disastrous.

Confidentiality and secrecy are adopted to avoid stigma. Proposed marital alliances tend to snap if the other party comes to know of mental illness of the boy or the girl.

Justice M Venkatachaliah, in his famous judgment 1988, In the (Rama Narain Gupta Vs Ms Rameshwari Gupta) observed that,

" All persons suffering from schizophrenia cannot be considered equally. Each case of schizophrenia should be viewed not only with a pure medical or legal perspective, but also a social and cultural perspective should be applied. The mere labeling as schizophrenia has no meaning.

"Schizophrenia is what Schizophrenia does".

In another Landmark Supreme Court Judgment (2013), Justice GS Singhvi and V Gopala Gowda, observed in the case of (Kollam Padma Latha Vs Kollam Chandra Sekhar)

"Wife can't be dumped on grounds of schizophrenia".

"Schizophrenia is a treatable, manageable disease, which can be put on par with hypertension and diabetes".

These notable judgments are very important in reducing the stigma and discrimination attached to the persons suffering from schizophrenia.

A sense of shame and disgrace can occur in a patient, who has apparently recovered from a bout of psychiatric illness.

Similarly, the prospect of lifelong medication stigmatizes and may lead to the threat of suicide. A few families wish that the mentally ill under their care are eliminated by nature and supplicate to the doctor if something could be done to terminate their lives. A mixture of feeling of helplessness, hopelessness, loss of morale, guilt, and a social stigma can create a dismal setting in which such expressions figure. Several methods are resorted to conceal clinical illness.

- Takes the medicines in his work spot and not at home
- Takes the tablets from the bottles with labels marked as vitamins, etc.
- Some girls are brought by without the knowledge of their husbands, when they come to parental homes. Not all are successful in these acts of hiding. Unfortunately, the prescription falls in their hands and are shown to their family doctor or someone else who point out these drugs are for mental illness.

FELT STIGMA (INTERNAL STIGMA)

The frequent bombardment of derogatory language such as 'mental', 'nutters', 'lunatics' and 'psycho', as well as the frequent use of unflattering and unrealistic imagery cannot help to engender good feelings in those with mental health problems. The first issue here is the felt experience and issue of self-stigmatization concerning how individuals come to reappraise their experience in light of media coverage. This is illustrated by Gilbert (2003) with regard to the process of external and internal shame. The external shame might include the feeling that 'others see me as unattractive', which results in a sense of internal shame in that 'I see myself as unattractive'. The shame and expectation of discrimination prevents people from talking about their experiences and discourages them from seeking help. An individual's concept of self is affected through stigma with enhanced feelings of hopelessness, low-self worth and increased/social withdrawal (Gray 2002). The prejudice and discrimination experienced can compound the distress felt and interfere further with personal coping skills already affected as a result of mental health problems (Johnstone 2001).

STIGMA AND NEGATIVE APPRAISAL

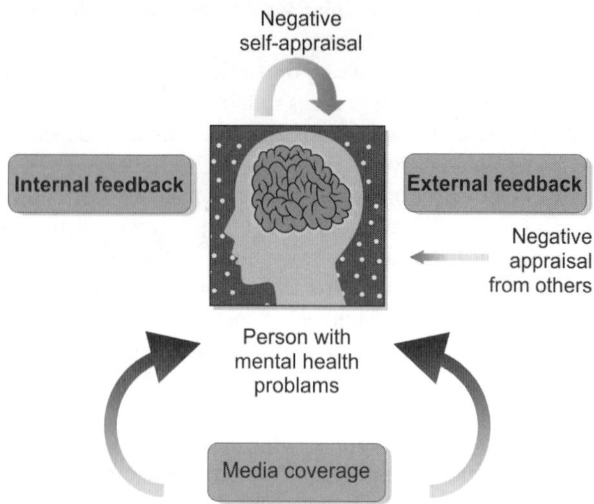

A number of those experiencing mental health problems indicate the extreme feelings of anxiety felt regarding their 'coming out'. Sayee (2000) states for some, this can be a liberating experience, yet for others, it can be hard to reconcile the different aspects of themselves such as competent researcher and mental health survivor. Certainly, the liberating process is reflected upon in a number of autobiographical accounts, as demonstrated by the footballer Tony Adams writing in the book "Addicted" about his coping with alcoholism and Maradona's, (the great football player) open statement about his drug addiction and further rehabilitation in a deaddiction center. The 'coming out' by notable individuals is in some cases greeted favorably by the public as exampled by Norwegian Prime Minister Mr. Bondevik's decision to take time off with depression, an action applauded by public and even his political opponents. Another notable example was the revelation by Princess Diana about her struggles with eating disorder, bulimia. This all plays a major role in reducing the sense and feeling of felt stigma experienced by those with mental health problems. What we learn about mental health issues is largely generated by what is picked up from the media (Philo 1996a). The media subsequently develop products that are regarded as appealing and reflecting the needs and interests of their audience.

A major problem affecting the mentally ill through the process of stigmatization is that of social exclusion.

COURTESY STIGMA

The power of stigma is such that it does not reside alone with the mentally ill, but can be widened to include others such as families, friends, and carers (Ostman and Kjellin in 2002). Stigma by association or 'courtesy stigma' relates to the problem, whereby the family of a 'mentally ill' individual may share some of the discredit of their stigmatized relative (Angermeyer, et al. 2003). The aspect of how stigma affects and envelopes others close to and involved with the mentally ill has been paid little attention by researchers. The concept of family burden has been looked at although not specifically with regards to the concept of stigma.

The level of our ignorance is such that it is safe to predict that much more time is necessary before we learn enough about schizophrenia to be able to prevent it. We can however provide care to people who suffer from schizophrenia and know what could enhance the probability that our treatment will be successful and that patients will find their place in society. We know what obstacles stand in the way of recovery and rehabilitation. Among these obstacles, undoubtedly, the most serious and difficult is the stigmatization of mental illness and of all those in contact with it—the sufferers, their families, the medications used for treatment, the institutions in which treatment is provided, staff in mental health institutions and even the sties on which they are located.

The stigma attached to mental illness and all that is related to it is the main obstacle to better mental health care and better quality of life of people who have the illness, of their families, of their communities and of health service staff that deals with psychiatric disorders. It is a basic component of the negative discrimination that people with mental illness experience every day. Stigma is pernicious and what is wore there are indications that despite advances of psychiatry and medicine, stigma continues to grow and has more and more often terrible consequences for patients and families.

THE VARIOUS CYCLE OF STIGMATIZATION

The model implies that a marker (a visible abnormality) that allows the identification of a person can be loaded with negative contents by association with previous knowledge, information obtained through the press, and memories of things seen in movies or heard in the community.

CYCLE OF STIGMATIZATION FOR THE INDIVIDUAL

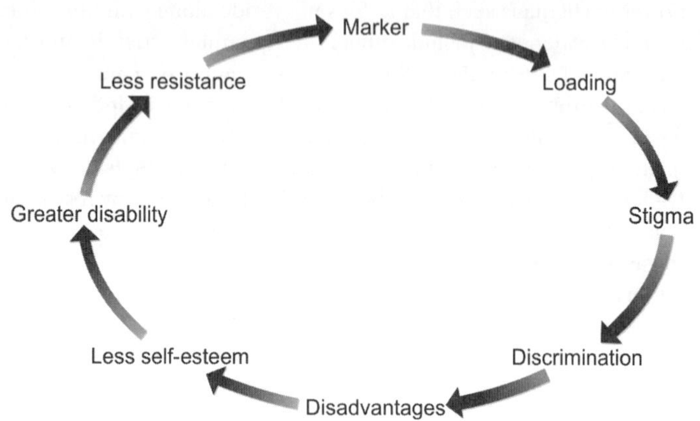

CYCLES OF STIGMATIZATION FOR THE FAMILY

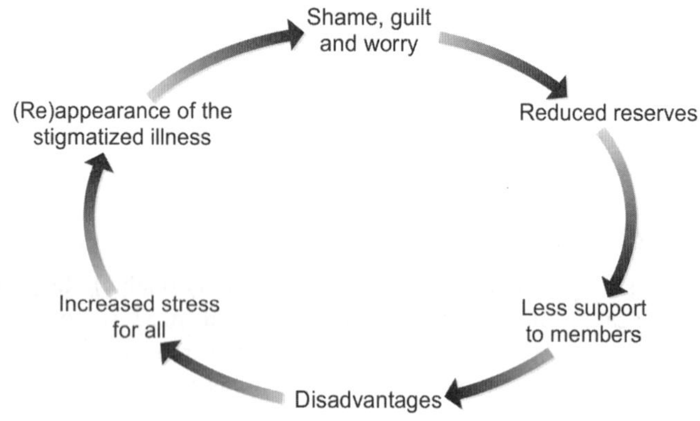

CYCLE OF STIGMATIZATION FOR MENTAL HEALTH SERVICES

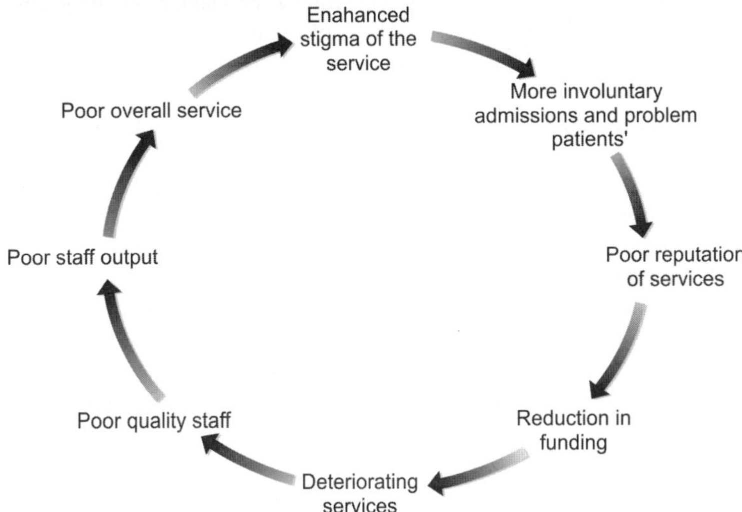

These cycles reinforce stereotypes, increase cynicism in members of the community, and further diminish hopes of those living with mental illness that things will improve.

These cycles of stigmatization are not isolated from each other. A family that has lost hope and self-esteem will find it more difficult to seek help and realize its right to help. This will not only worsen the situation, but also contribute to the perception of weakness of the family and all of its members, and lessen their ability to become active participants along with the health care professionals in the recovery of the family member with schizophrenia.

These interrelated cycles of stigma and discrimination because of mental illness illustrate specific points for intervention. The next question becomes one of how finally focused the interventions should be:

- Stigma becomes one of the important factors from patient's side, which affect mental health services in rural areas
- Diagnoses of mental disorders carry implications that are different from diagnoses of purely somatic illnesses, in part because of the societal stigma attached to mental illnesses. This stigma has ancient roots. Human mankind attaches great power to the mind, but finds it deeply mysterious. One of the worst fears is the loss of meaningful connections, decision making ability and intellectual capacity (Trad, 1991)
- Ship of Fools' approach (stigmatization of the population). Captain of some vessels would accept deranged persons for a fee and ferry them

about the water ways of Europe, sometimes to be left in an isolated city, sometimes consigned to permanent life on the ships and usually to be the object of amusement and ridicule when such a ship came to the port

- These traditions form the fear and misunderstanding about mental illnesses and its cause that still persists as a stigma that may keep sufferers from seeking help
- It has been suggested that stigma may be less severe in Asian and African countries, but still a study carried out in India within the stigma program of the WPA, reported that two-thirds of the respondents had suffered discrimination. Women and people living in urban areas were more stigmatized
- Men experienced greater discrimination in the job area, where as women experienced more problems in the family and social areas. In the family area, subtle discrimination in the form of decreased love, avoidance, rejection, distance and excessive caution were frequently reported
- In Ethiopia, among relatives of people with severe mental disorder, 75% reported that they had experienced stigma due to the presence of mental illness in their family and 37% wanted to cancel the fact that the relative was ill
- In a large survey carried out in China, among people with schizophrenia and their family members, are half of the respondents reported they had felt significantly stigmatized and levels of stigma were found to be higher in urban areas
- Stigmatization of people with mental disorders has been reported to be rare in Islamic Countries
- In countries like Turkey, Mongolia and South Africa, the view that "weakness", "laziness", or "lack of will-power" contribute to the development of mental disorders, has been reported
- Stigmatization of people with mental disorders may result in public avoidance, systematic discrimination and reduced help seeking behavior
- Although most countries have some provision for disability benefits, people with mental illness, are often specific excluded from entilements, this barrier has recently been removed in India and apart from mental retardation, mental disorders have also been included as one of the six disabilities in the Disabilities Act.

Moreover, mental disorders are frequently not considered in social and private insurance schemes for health care.

Shame is reported to be one of the main barriers from seeking help for mental disorders in both developed and developing countries.

Selected International Research Findings on Stigma

1. "In contrast to adults, adolescence reported that contact lead to more discrimination"—Corrigan, et al. 2005.
2. "Close association between high expressed emotion and perceived effect of stigma"—Phillips, et al. 2002.
3. "Serious films out-numbered by exploitation/horror films"—Schneider, 1987.
4. "Newspaper portray mentally ill in a negative fashion"—Day, et al. 1986.
5. "Most employers were cautious and hesitant to employ persons with mental illness than persons with physical illness"—Manning and White, 1995.
6. "Education yields some positive benefits, contact with patients is the greatest results, protest yielded no improvement"—Corrigan, et al. 2001 and 2002.
7. "Both stigma acceptance and stigma avoidance are irritating and energy consuming processes"—Katsching, 2000.
8. "Nature of the Psychiatrists job itself can be stigmatizing. So can the side effects of medications prescribed"—Hotopf, 2000.

Selected summary of Indian Studies on Stigma

1. "Public fears and rejects mentally ill; rural population more tolerant"—Neki, 1966.
2. "Misconception, superstition and ignorance; viewing mental illness as visitation of the evil spirits"—Dube, 1970.
3. "Majority had positive attitudes; two-thirds against marital alliance to a family, with a history of mental illness"—Verghese and Baig, 1974.
4. "Pessimistic community attitudes; preferred modern health services and later returning to traditional healers"—Wig, et al. 1980.
5. "Marriage, dread of rejection from neighbors, concealing the illness, being a female and younger age of caregiver and patient were worst stigmatizing"
   "Families believing in the supernatural causations of illness less likely"
   "Women separated husbands—but not legally concerned about their future, being a burden to ageing parents"—Thara and Srinivasan, 2000, 2001, 2003.
6. "Awareness more among literates and urban; females felt sexual harassment as a consequence of stigma; in general, stigma was due to emphasis on heredity as a cause, fear of violence and need for life-long care"—Murthy, et al. 2005.
7. "Stigma and discrimination were most experienced during the acute phase of the illness."

"Lack of awareness, difficulty in working, and attribution of a supernatural cause were the other variables, apart from socially unacceptable behavior create stigma".

"Experience of ridicule, shame, and discrimination was more in the rural sample".

"Concerns about disclosure and the impact of the illness had on the self-esteem of the caregivers and family members figured as distressing stigma related perceptions"—Loganathan S and Murthy RS, 2008.

8. "The perception and the attitude of the society towards the mentally ill has not changed much overtime. The recent incidents like mentally ill patients being chained and getting burnt alive at Erwadi (Tamil Nadu) reminds as how such patients were treated and ostracized in our society. The stigma is a major impediment in the treatment and integration of the mentally ill in the society"—H Khurana, et al. 2006.
9 "Rural Indians showed more stigmatizing attitudes towards severe mental illness. Urban Indians reported a more liberal and tolerant attitude, but were also of more excluding of those with mental illness at work."—Jadhav S, et al. 2007.

STIGMA AND SPECIFIC MENTAL HEALTH PROBLEMS (OTHER THAN SCHIZOPHRENIA)

ECT and stigma: Though ECT is one of the most effective types of treatment, particularly for depression with suicidal ideas, it is portrayed as a much malignant treatment particularly by human rights activists and to the lay media. This is mainly because of differing points of view and misunderstanding about the scientific basis of the treatment. Many patients and relatives still think that

- ECT is given as a punishment
- ECT induces memory loss
- Causes brain damage, sometimes permanent.

SUICIDE BEHAVIOR

Until recently, there were religious sanctions against suicide and stigma prevails in Islamic Countries too with the result the suicides are grossly under reported: stigma afflicts those who attempt suicide and also the surviving members of completed suicide. The suicide attempters suffer from additional dose of stigma being legally involved. The laws need to be revised in this respect. Section 309 IPC considers attempted suicide is still a criminal behavior. It is a cry for help, an act of despair, and a disease of hope which need psychological care and should not be labeled as a criminal behavior.

Although suicide is regarded as a problem everywhere, associated stigma and condemnation are not absolute. Culturally sanctioned suicides in response to humiliation, widowhood, or in order to manipulate political events, acute poverty indicate that these acts convey meanings and consequences. Suicides related to political events, Mandal's Phenomenon and farmers suicide in India fall under this category. At times, these suicides are glorified.

Stigma of psychiatric evaluation or assignments of psychiatric diagnoses form an important barrier to psychiatric care as the end life.

STIGMA AND MOOD DISORDERS

Stigmatizing attitudes towards people with mood disorders are widespread in the general public even among health care providers including mental health professionals.

There exists little research on stigmatizing attitudes towards people with mood disorders. Most of the literature on the stigma towards people with mental illness relates to people with more severe disorders such as schizophrenia. When research has been done on mood disorders, the focus has been on perceived stigma and self stigma. No up-to-date research exists on discrimination experienced by people with mood disorders and very little research exists on interventions designed to decrease stigmatizing attitudes towards them.

High stigma surrounding childhood disorders poses unique access barriers for youth and their families and merits further study to identify ways to combat their harmful perception.

MEDIA AND STIGMA

"In this connection, it is important to refer to the unfortunate role which media in our country like cinema, TV, or press, has played in perpetuating the prejudice against mental disorders. Mental illness is always shown as something to ridicule, something is laugh at, or something which is bizarre, disgusting or frightening.

Of late, there have been some excellent depictions of mental illness, like the blockbuster Tamil movie "Chandramukhi" and "Annian". It is refreshing to note that these movies have been well researched and psychiatrist is portrayed in a positive way.

Selection of media types features some of the more prominently negative characteristics or examples portrayed. The sources covered are those of film, TV, internet, press and literature.

Films like Tare Zameen Par, which reveals the positive aspects of dyslexia and Tamil movie like Haridas depicts the positive aspects of autism.

The Beautiful Mind, the Oscar Award winner movie, which depicts the importance of caregiving and the intellectual ability and the capacity of the persons suffering from schizophrenia inspite of the disease are vividly picturized.

Negative representation is the predominant message being relayed and can be found in all media source types from the print media, film, TV and radio, through to the new electronic media. The degree to which stigmatizing mental health imagery is reflected in the media is outlined in a number of current publications and reports. SIEFF (2003) identifies, the frequently negative frames deployed by the mass media contribute towards the persistence of the public's negative attitudes regarding the mentally ill. This sets up a cyclical relationship whereby negative perceptions are reinforced. Mental disorder and mental ill health stand worldwide as being one of the most stigmatized of all human conditions. There has been a shift over recent years towards a greater social awareness, enhanced advocacy and a greater 'voice' being developed regarding those experiencing mental health problems.

Mental illness has always been the substrate for comedy, sex, violence and crime, which inturn strengthens the various misconceptions in the minds of the public about mental illness and thereby increases the stigma.

Peter Lorre who, because of his distinctively odd appearance, was chosen to play the deranged killer in a succession of films or the wide gulf between wellness and illness (Jim Carrey's Jekyll and Hyde Portrayal in Me, Myself and Irene). These characterizations help to perpetuate the social myth that we can spot those with mental health problems by their appearance and behavior alone. It serves to further distance those with mental health problems from others and fits Wahl's (1995) classification of a 'breed apart.'

The stereotypical association between violence and mental health issues is found in profilic quantity within the medium of film.

A key feature evoking criticism about the film portrayals of mental illness relates to the huge number of inaccuracies or misrepresentation being shown. One film in particular that was greeted of Me, Myself and Irene. This movie enormously featured the main character's split personality with the good self being manifested in his mentally well part and the bad self represented by his mentally ill one. The fact that this film proved such a huge success at the box office is a depressing one given the number of people exposed to such negative and misleading facts about mental illness. The scale of misrepresentation within the cinema is huge and even extends towards the 'based upon a true story' type of film.

This was clearly built up and exaggerated for the benefit of offering the viewer cues for dramatic engagement.

The story presented to the audience therefore can be regarded as a construct of the director, scriptwriter and film crew, with commercial and artistic considerations having a major say in how the person's story is told.

There are many examples whereby those with mental health problems are grossly misrepresented. Negative characterization of mentally ill characters being used in Televison programs especially in serials. It is clearly the case that madness is attractive to viewers and certainly something that adds extra drama or impact to products.

There are many chat shows and reality TV formats in television today. The chat shows range from the sensitive and informative to the grossly exploitative and abusive. There is also an important function here for viewers who can engage in a form of vicarious therapy, connecting with and feeling supported by the experience shared by participants. All of this aptly sumps up Woods' (2002) statement about reality TV as a form of mass voyeurism where a person's dignity no longer matters.

One of the biggest strengths of the internet also provides one of its main problems in that the easy availability and access of vast stores of information causes problems for consumers in terms of sifting through and selecting what is relevant. Some of the valid and worthy material accessible online remains unseen or unappreciated by many of those at whom it is targeted.

A brief search of the internet can prove a bewildering and confusing process as a fair degree of the information accessed appears contrary to that found on other more authoritative sites. It is therefore very worrying to reflect upon those internet sites which advocate self-harmful behaviors and sanitize the very real and distressing nature of suicide through their use of terms such as 'self-deliverance'.

Nowadays, many patients and the caregivers go to internet and verify our prescriptions where all the side effects including the rarest are given. On seeing this, they are reluctant to continue this medication.

WAYS TO MINIMIZE STIGMA

Stigma and discrimination experienced by persons suffering from mental illness is a universal phenomenon. Unlike other medical conditions, it is recognized as an important barrier in countries rich and poor, big and small and in countries with well developed mental health services and those with limited services (World Health Organization, 2001).

Mental health professionals are aware of the harmful effect of stigma against mental illness. It interferes at every stage in the diagnosis, treatment and rehabilitation of all types of mental disorders, and even forces people to avoid seeking psychiatric help. Fighting this stigma can improve the outcome of the disease, and allow the patients to make use of the new modalities of treatment that bring new hope to them. (Wig, 1997).

The stigma centers mainly around heredity of mental illness and socially unacceptable behavior like aggression, disinhibition and related behaviors (Orley and Wing, 1979) in India and other developing countries.

Increasing knowledge in the community about mental disorders is an important means of fighting stigma.

Secondly, organizing essential psychiatric services to cover the total population is a priority in developing countries.

Thirdly, mental health professionals have a very important role in fighting the stigma, since they will be the focal point for the community to find alternatives.

Fourthly, the media presentation of mental disorders should be changed.

Fifthly, mental health professionals can learn from experiences of fighting stigma from other stigmatizing medical conditions like cancer and AIDS.

We have identified various stigma related issues. Therefore, we can focus our efforts to make the situation better.

In Japan, the nomenclature of the term for schizophrenia was changed, which literally mean, "Integration Dysfunction Syndrome" in 2002 to minimize the stigma attached to mental illness.

In order to reduce stigma against psychiatry, we need to work with other areas beyond our expertise. When we make helpful service beyond psychiatry, people in other areas can appreciate us. What is needed? We need to provide our expertize in form of consultation and collaboration.

In addition to the ongoing projects like research on stigma against psychiatric illness or psychiatrists/psychiatry, physicians, other specialists, and general practitioners should be sensitized about the stigma attached to mental illness and create awareness to minimize such stigma.

We cannot expect people in other areas to understand psychiatric or even mental health terminologies. What we need to learn is their terminologies and the method how we can translate our expertize in their language and show seeable and understandable results according to their criteria. Then we can reduce stigma without fight. Consultation and collaboration are the key phrases of the movement against stigma in countries like Japan.

The Mental Health First Aid (MHFA) program launched in the West was originally designed to train members of public with the aim to enhance their mental health literacy and skills to help people in mental health crisis before professional help is available. The effectiveness of the program has been empirically demonstrated.

The main approach was "To dispel misconception and superstition about mental illness, to clarify the doubts of patients and caregivers, to demystify mental disorder and try to reduce the stigma attached to mental disorders and their treatment.

Mental health education should impart the following messages:

1. Mental health and physical health are truly inseparable and they influence each other in a complex and profound way.
2. Mental disorders are like any other physical disorders like diabetes mellitus and hypertension. Mental disorders are disorders of the functioning of brain in addition to the psychosocial adverse effects.

Stigma is difficult to overcome and the affected ones cope with them variously:

1. To consider mental illness on par with physical illness and informing the public that any physical disease like diabetes, high blood pressure, stomach ulcer, etc. has had some influence.
2. Setting up psychiatric departments in general hospitals may overcome the stigma of going to mental hospitals.
3. Giving a physical diagnosis like neurasthenia rather than depression in general practice seems to be more acceptable and less stigmatizing as reported in the Chinese culture. The word "Nerve" is more acceptable and respectable than "mental" or "psychiatry".
4. The term "Lunatic Asylum" had been changed "mental hospitals" which again recalled as "Institute of Mental Health or Human Behavior, but the question is do they exist. "Mind is the Agent of Change". Public education should bring an awareness of mental disorders or else education becomes targetless.

Internationally, fighting stigma is identified as the final obstacle to better mental health care (Sartorius, 1997). The President of India, in February 2004, called for a fight against stigma and discrimination against mentally ill persons. (The Hindu, 2004) and gave this specific pledge to young people. " I will always be a friend of the mentally and physically-challenged, including people with schizophrenia, and will work hard to make them feel normal".

International bodies like World Psychiatric Association, Royal College of Psychiatrists, World Health Organization have become involved to design and prepare materials to increase awareness of the public health, materials to increase awareness of the public health importance of this disease and helping to mitigate stigma and discrimination linked to it. The program is addressed to the families and patients, mental health workers working with the mentally ill besides community leaders, general practitioners and the general public.

That stigma exists and that it is pernicious is gradually becoming accepted (Link, et al. 1992). This growth of awareness is however only rarely accompanied by the commitment or at least willingness to do something about diminishing stigma and its consequences.

The reasons given for inaction by mental health workers (and by others who should be concerned with stigma) are varied. Some say that they are too busy, linked to mental illness is not very different from stigma attached to other illnesses and therefore only a comprehensive program, which is beyond their reach can make sense.

The international campaigns against stigma and discrimination of mental illness:

1. World Psychiatric Association (WPA) (1996) launched the "Open The Doors" initiative to increase awareness and knowledge of the nature of schizophrenia and treatment options.
   Understanding the pernicious impact of stigma on patients, their families and the health staff and institutions providing treatment and care, the World Psychiatric Association (WPA), initiated a Global Program Against Stigma and Discrimination, or at least diminishing its consequences.
   The program, initiated in 1996, grew rapidly and was soon designated by the WPA as one of its institutional programs.
   The program has received support from country authorities, psychiatric associations, patient and family associations, a variety of health institutions and from the health industry and one of its central aims is to become an integral part of everyday health services.
2. The World Health Day 2001 and The World Health Report 2001 to Mental Health, the WHO stated that "mental illness was ignored and mental health is essential to the overall wellbeing of the individuals". The WHO theme for 2001 was "Stop Exclusion. Dare To Care".
3. The American Psychiatric Association (1997) approved of a position statement on discrimination against persons with previous psychiatric treatment to facilitate their full participations in society.
4. In the UK, the Royal College of Psychiatrists and the Royal College of GP's launched a "Defeat Depression Campaign" in 1992.
5. "Changing Minds" organized by the Royal College of Psychiatrists in 2000 imparted information to the public so as to dispel myths and stereotypes about those with mental illness.

The World Psychiatric Association undertook a program to address the stigma and discrimination because of schizophrenia.

The group agreed to three guiding principles for the program.

- To survey individuals living with the illness and their family members about the experience of stigma and discrimination, and where possible encourage their active participation
- To encourage the participation of individuals throughout the community whether in health care, government or private enterprise—everyone was welcome;
- To ensure this was a long-term effort, rather than a brief campaign.

The first International Conference on the stigma and discrimination because of schizophrenia was held in Leipzig, Germany in 2001. In 2002, further findings were presented at the WPA Congress in Yokohama, Japan.

Strategies for addressing stigmatization of people with mental disorders have been subdivided into three groups:

1. Protest.
2. Education.
3. Contact.

Protest campaigns may be effective in reducing stigmatizing behaviors to same extent against people like mental disorders. Education promotes a better understanding and educated people may be less likely to endorse stigma and discrimination. An inverse relationship exists between having contact with a person with mental illness and endorsing stigmatizing behaviors, has been documented.

Advantages of treatment guidelines to reduce stigma: stigma and its effects on persons suffering from mental disorders, their families and treatment continue to be a major challenge. That mental illnesses are real and diagnosable are explicitly demonstrated by guidelines.

Indian mental health professionals have conducted many studies on the attitude of general public towards mental illness and in the process have developed special psychological research instruments suitable for attitudinal studies in our population. In this connection, one may refer to the development of culture specific valid and reliable questionnaires (Prabhu 1983) and development of socioculturally relevant vignettes stories (Malhotra and Wig, 1975) and pictures (Murthy, et al. 1985). In an excellent review of public attitude towards mental illness in India, Prabhu, et al. concluded that. "'The general trend of the studies carried out in India indicate that the lay public including the educated urban groups, are largely uninformed about the various aspects of mental health. The mentally ill are perceived as aggressive, violent and dangerous. There is a lack of awareness about the available facilities to treat the mentally ill and a pervasive defeatism exists about the possible outcome after therapy. There is a tendency to maintain social distance from the mentally ill and to reject them" (Prabhu, et al. 1984).

CONCLUSION

Stigma has been the topic of research and discussion for decades. Stigma encompasses the negative stereotypes and prejudicial beliefs that people may hold, as well as discriminatory or inequitable practices that may result. The stigma of mental illness, although, more often related to context than to a person's appearance, remains a powerful negative attribute in all social relations.

Adverse attitudes to mental illnesses are found in all societies of the world. Latest researches have revealed that psychiatry, psychiatrists, mental health professionals, and the mentally ill patients are affected by negative prejudices and the cultural stereotypes of the general public.

There has been a major effort in recent years to actively fight against stigmatizing attitudes and discrimination, mainly through education via public policy, media, and educational packages for schools and workplaces.

Anecdotal evidence suggests that stigmatizing attitudes may have decreased. Society, however, is still a long way from accepting mental disorders to the extent in which physical health problems are accepted. Stigma affects the quality of life of people with mental disorders in many ways. People who develop mental disorders and have high levels of stigmatizing attitudes may delay or avoid help seeking or may not comply with the treatment recommendations. Disclosing diagnosis of mental disorder may lead to discrimination, harassment, or avoidance of social contact by others who have stigmatizing attitudes.

The following are some suggestions to minimize stigma towards mental disorders:

1. Awareness and mental health education programs to public through various methods.
2. Sensitizing the other share holders like advocates, judiciary, police officials, administrators and also politicians (if possible) to create awareness and to reduce misconceptions about mental illness.
3. Sensitizing media people to portray the positive aspects of mental health care aspects and to some extent minimize the negative aspects in their creations.
4. Integrating mental health care with the general health care with more effective ways of introducing DMHP Programs.
5. Inclusion of psychiatry as an exam subject for UG medical studies.
6. Creating awareness and sensitizing knowledge about severe and common mental disorders and the positive approach to initiate and maintain psychiatric treatment to general practitioners, physicians and other specialists is essential. Very often, our non-psychiatric collegues are the main reasons for our patient's negative attitude to initiate or maintain psychiatric treatment.

Above all, we should have the insight that stigma surrounding mental disorders cannot be eradicated overnight. It will take a long time even if we initiate our active efforts now.

Fighting stigma is not a 100-meter dash, but a marathon, and the efforts should be to plan for long-term programs.

"It is better to light a candle rather than Cursing the Darkness".

Appendices

APPENDIX 1: COMPARISON OF SOME COMMON PSYCHIATRIC DISORDERS

Neurosis vs Psychosis

Neurosis	Psychosis
1. Mild mental disturbance	Major mental disturbance
2. Patient frequently talks about his/her symptoms and wants to get cured (insight present)	The psychotic often denies that there is anything wrong with him (insight absent)
3. The person does not lose contact with reality	The psychotic has lost contact with reality
4. Personality is well preserved even after years of illness	Personality may be disorganized with or deteriorated
5. The person continues to function socially and on the job	Social life and occupation often get disrupted
6. Does not harm himself seriously or harm others	May harm himself or others
7. Outcome (prognosis) is generally good	Outcome not so good in some psychotic disorders

Major Depression vs Dysthmic Depression (Endogenous vs Neurotic Depression)

Major depression	Dysthmic depression
Primary disturbance in the structure and function of the brain and nervous system	Severe, prolonged stress, unresolved conflicts, chronic anxiety, fears, anger
Rapid and without apparent cause	Gradual
Restlessness and agitation, or psychomotor retardation severe; tends to be worse in morning and better in evening	Mixed, mild to severe unpredictable mood; usually optimistic in morning and depressed in evening

Contd...

Contd...

Major depression	Dysthmic depression
Insomnia after being awakened	Easily awakened, but goes back to deep sleep in the morning
Early morning awakening	Sleep initiation delayed
Anorexia, leading to weight loss	Varied (anorexia leading to compulsive eating)
Chronically tired; needs support at all times	Occasional energy bursts
Very low spirits	Fluctuates from high to low
Intense fear of being alone	Multiple fears about the present and future
Totally indecisive	Okay on minor decisions; indecisive on important decisions
Paranoid, self-depreciatory delusions, distorted judgment	No psychotic symptoms

Epilepsy vs Hysterical Fit

	Epilepsy	Hysterical fit
1. History of fall and injury	Present	Absent
2. Fits when alone/during sleep	Yes	No
3. Every fit same as the other	Yes	No
4. Movement of the limbs	Regular	Irregular
5. Tongue bite	Yes	No
6. Incontinence of urine and feces	Yes	No
7. Inducing an attack by strong suggestion	Not possible	Possible
8. Pupils and plantar reflex during an attack	Dilated pupils Upgoing plantars	Normal

Delirium vs Dementia

Delirium	Dementia
1. Acute onset	Insidious onset
2. Presence of disorientation, anxiety, poor attention	Disturbed memory, personality deterioration

Contd...

Contd...

Delirium	Dementia
3. Clouding of consciousness, e.g. drowsiness	Clear consciousness
4. Perceptual abnormalities are common (illusions, hallucinations)	Global impairment of cerebral function
5. Fluctuating course with lucid intervals	Progressive course
6. Reversible	Mostly irreversible

Attempted Suicide vs Suicide

Attempted suicide	Suicide
1. Only an attempt person is alive	A completed act; person is dead
2. More common in females	More common among males
3. Physical illness—No obvious association	Probable association
4. Main psychiatric diagnosis—Adjustment disorder, depression hysteria, situation reaction, alcoholism, drug dependence	Mood disorder, alcoholism, drug dependence and schizophrenia
5. Triggering factors—Psychosocial factors more common	Biological factors more common

APPENDIX II: RATING SCALES IN PSYCHIATRY

Screening Test for Alcoholism—'CAGE'

C Have you ever felt you ought to *cut* down on your drinking?
A Have people *annoyed* you by criticizing your drinking?
G Have you ever felt bad or *guilty* about your drinking?
E Have you ever had a drink first thing in the morning to steady your nerves or get rid of a hangover (*eye opener*)?

If you get positive replies to any two of these questions, it is worth taking a proper drinking history.

A Short Mood Scale

Anxiety

1. Have you felt keyed-up, and on the edge?
2. Have you been worrying a lot?
3. Have you been irritable?
4. Have you had difficulty in relaxing?

If 'Yes' to any two of above, go on to:

5. Have you been sleeping poorly?
6. Have you had headaches (or neckaches or tightness in head)?
7. Have you had dizziness, trembling, sweating, diarrhea, frequent urination, tingling, etc. (autonomic anxiety)?
8. Have you been worried about health?
9. Have you had difficulty in falling asleep?

Depression

1. Do you feel lacking in energy?
2. Are you losing interest in things?
3. Have you lost confidence in yourself?
4. Have you ever felt hopeless?

If 'Yes' to anyone of above, go on to:

5. Are you unable to concentrate?
6. Have you lost weight? (due to poor appetite)
7. Do you wake up early?
8. Do you feel you are slowing down?
9. Have you felt worse in mornings?

   1 Point for each positive answer.

   Anxiety states usually score at least 5 on A, depressive at least 3 on B.

Assessment of Suicidal Risk

Recent Self-Poisoning (or Injury)

Objective: What drugs were taken? How much? When? Where? Who else was there? Whom did the patient inform? What were the arrangements to avoid being found?

Subjective: Patient's statement about purpose. Knowledge concerning drugs taken. Attitude to being alive now.

Illness Associated with Increased Risk

Does history and mental examination suggest evidence of:

- Depressive illness
- Alcoholism, other addictions
- Schizophrenia
- Dementia
- Epilepsy
- Antisocial personality
- Chronic, painful physical disease.

What does the patient say about suicidal thoughts and intentions now?

Demographic and Social Data

- Age, sex, social class, occupation, marital status.
- Social isolation
- Unemployment
- Bereavement.

Remember: The best predictor of suicide is an episode of self-poisoning.

Ward Behavior Scales (Wing's)

Please consider the patient's behavior during the past week only, even if it was not typical of his or her usual condition.

There are three items in each section. If one of the items describes behavior which has occurred in the past week, please, place a tick against it in the column on the right. There should be only one tick for each section. Please read all three items before making your choice.

Item I: Slowness of Movement

(2) Usually extremely slow to move, e.g. took very much longer over a meal, or dressing, or walking across the ward, than other patients.

(1) Showed periods of extreme slowness of movement as in (2), but at other times was not slow to move.

(0) Speed of movement normal.

Item 2: Under-Activity

(2) Stood or sat in one place all the time, with little movement. Even with encouragement, was very difficult to get moving.
(1) Showed periods of extreme under-activity as in (2), but at other times was not under-active.
(0) Showed no marked under-activity.

Item 3: Over-Activity

(2) Usually extremely over-active or restless, e.g. paced rapidly up and down, became excited, talked or sang loudly or wildly, etc.
(1) Showed periods of extreme over-activity as in (2), but at other times was not over-active.
(0) Showed no marked over-activity.

Item 4: Conversation

(2) Was mute or almost mute.
(1) Said a few words, e.g. in reply to questions, but was usually silent.
(0) Ordinary conversation.

Item 5: Social Withdrawal

(2) Never mixed socially with anyone, even when encouraged to do so.
(1) Was socially withdrawn and solitary, but would mix a little with others if encouraged to do so.
(0) Normal social mixing.

Item 6: Leisure Interests

(2) Showed no interest in anything. Did not watch television, read newspapers, play games, etc. even when encouraged to do so.
(1) Showed very little interest, but could be persuaded to watch television, read newspapers, join in games, etc. for a while.
(0) Showed normal spontaneous interest.

Item 7: Laughing and Talking to Self

(2) Frequent episodes (once a day or more often) of laughing or talking out loud-not just constant smiling.
(1) Occasional episodes of laughing or talking out loud, but these did not occur every day.
(0) No such episodes noted.

Item 8: Posturing and Mannerisms

(2) Adopted odd or uncomfortable postures, or made bizarre movements everyday.
(1) Behaved as in (2), but less often than everyday.
(0) No such behavior seen.

Item 9: Threatening or Violent Behavior

(2) Struck someone, or destroyed something (e.g. clothing, window, crockery, etc.)
(1) Was threatening in manner, or verbally abusive, but did not strike anyone.
(0) No such behavior seen.

Item 10: Personal Hygiene

(2) Was incontinent on atleast one occasion during the week.
(1) Needed raising at night or escorting to lavatory during the day, in case of incontinence, but was not actually incontinent when this was done.
(0) Needed no escorting or raising and was not incontinent.

Item 11: Personal Appearance

(2) Needed to be shaved (if male), washed or dressed fully at least once during the week.
(1) Could shave, dress and wash, but needed supervision with tie, buttons, etc. or would be slovenly in appearance.
(0) Needed no supervision of this kind. Maintained reasonably neat appearance without prompting.

Item 12: Behavior at Meal Times

(2) Needed spoon feeding at least once during the week.
(1) Did not require spoon-feeding, but had to wear bib, or needed supervision because of faulty table manners.
(0) Normal Behavior at meal times.

Nurses Observation Scale for Inpatient Evaluation (NOSIE)

A behavior rating scale to be filled by the nurse after observation of inpatient in the chronic mentally ill ward. This rating scale consists of 30 items. Symptoms or behavior is scored from 0 (never) to 4 (always) experience and minimal training for the nurse is sufficient to rate this scale. This rating scale is used much in evaluating inpatients, especially schizophrenics. This scale can also be used to assess geriatric patients. This scale can assess the following areas: social interest, social competence, personal hygiene, irritability psychomotor retardation, manifest psychosis and sadness.

Direction

In the following pages, you are asked to rate the behavior of the patient. There are 80 items, which cover a wide range of activities. You are to base your ratings on the patient's behavior during the last three days only. For each item you are to estimate whether in the last days the description of the patient's behavior was true:

0 Never
1 Sometimes
2 Often
3 Usually
4 Always

Indicate your choice by placing a circle around the correct number before each item.

0	1	2	3	4	1. Is sloppy
0	1	2	3	4	2. Is impatient
0	1	2	3	4	3. Accuses others of wanting to hurt him
0	1	2	3	4	4. Ignores the activities around him
0	1	2	3	4	5. Cries
0	1	2	3	4	6. Demands attention of the doctors
0	1	2	3	4	7. Has temper tantrums
0	1	2	3	4	8. Resists suggestions and requests
0	1	2	3	4	9. Shouts and yell
0	1	2	3	4	10. Is excited and noisy
0	1	2	3	4	11. Gets along with other patients
0	1	2	3	4	12. Talks freely with volunteer workers or other visitors
0	1	2	3	4	13. Shows curiosity and interest in activities around him
0	1	2	3	4	14. Keeps busy during the day
0	1	2	3	4	15. Conforms to the hospital routine
0	1	2	3	4	16. Is cheerful and optimistic
0	1	2	3	4	17. Hoards things (carries things hidden in paper bags, hides things under bed, etc.)
0	1	2	3	4	18. Hits others
0	1	2	3	4	19. Shaves himself
0	1	2	3	4	20. Speaks in short phrases only (3 or 4 words at a time)

0	1	2	3	4	21. Looks sad
0	1	2	3	4	22. Needs help in dressing
0	1	2	3	4	23. Needs help in using the toilet
0	1	2	3	4	24. Helps out when asked
0	1	2	3	4	25. Plays cards with others
0	1	2	3	4	26. Sits unless directed into activity
0	1	2	3	4	27. Knows where he is
0	1	2	3	4	28. Cooperates with other people
0	1	2	3	4	29. Talks about himself
0	1	2	3	4	30. Stays by himself
0	1	2	3	4	31. Is hesitant and uncertain in making up his mind
0	1	2	3	4	32. Jokes with others
0	1	2	3	4	33. Gets angry or annoyed easily
0	1	2	3	4	34. Wets or soils his clothes or bedding
0	1	2	3	4	35. Asks for a pass to leave the hospital
0	1	2	3	4	36. Talks about happenings in the ward
0	1	2	3	4	37. Answers when spoken to
0	1	2	3	4	38. Hears things that are not there
0	1	2	3	4	39. Seems content and satisfied
0	1	2	3	4	40. Keeps his clothes neat and clean
0	1	2	3	4	41. Takes part in back and forth conversation
0	1	2	3	4	42. Complains about the food and care
0	1	2	3	4	43. Tries to be friendly with others
0	1	2	3	4	44. Becomes easily upset if something does not suit him
0	1	2	3	4	45. Assumes strange expressions, postures or movements
0	1	2	3	4	46. Refuses to do the ordinary things expected of him
0	1	2	3	4	47. Is irritable and grouchy
0	1	2	3	4	48. Has trouble remembering
0	1	2	3	4	49. Makes his own bed
0	1	2	3	4	50. Refuses to speak
0	1	2	3	4	51. Can be drawn into conversation
0	1	2	3	4	52. Laughs or smiles at funny comments or events
0	1	2	3	4	53. Volunteers to help out around the ward
0	1	2	3	4	54. Claims that he is being controlled by people or unusual forces
0	1	2	3	4	55. Is messy in his eating habits

0	1	2	3	4	56. Starts conversations with others
0	1	2	3	4	57. Says he feels blue or depressed
0	1	2	3	4	58. Combs his hair
0	1	2	3	4	59. Talks about his interests
0	1	2	3	4	60. Takes part in recreation
0	1	2	3	4	61. Sees things that are not there
0	1	2	3	4	62. Is friendly with someone in the ward
0	1	2	3	4	63. Has unusual speech (mixes up words, makes up new words, repeats sounds, words, or phrases in a meaningless or mechanical manner)
0	1	2	3	4	64. Shows inappropriate feeling or lack of feeling
0	1	2	3	4	65. Reads newspapers and magazines
0	1	2	3	4	66. Has to be reminded what to do
0	1	2	3	4	67. Sleeps, unless directed into activity
0	1	2	3	4	68. Says that he is no good
0	1	2	3	4	69. Has to be told to follow hospital routine
0	1	2	3	4	70. Seems to enjoy life
0	1	2	3	4	71. Pays attention when spoken to
0	1	2	3	4	72. Washes himself
0	1	2	3	4	73. Has difficulty completing even simple talks on his own
0	1	2	3	4	74. Is alert and attentive
0	1	2	3	4	75. Talks, mutters or mumbles to himself
0	1	2	3	4	76. Appears confused or puzzled
0	1	2	3	4	77. Is slow moving and sluggish
0	1	2	3	4	78. Giggles or smiles to himself without any apparent reason
0	1	2	3	4	79. Quick to fly off the handle
0	1	2	3	4	80. Keeps himself neat and clean

APPENDIX III: MENTAL HOSPITALS IN INDIA

States	Number of hospitals
Andhra Pradesh	2
Assam	1
Bihar	3
Goa	1
Gujarat	6
Jammu & Kashmir	2
Karnataka	2
Kerala	3
Madhya Pradesh	2
Maharashtra	5
Nagaland	1
Orissa	1
Punjab	1
Rajasthan	2
Tamil Nadu	1
Uttar Pradesh	4
West Bengal	7
Delhi	1
Total	45

List of Institutions Having Specialized Treatment Facilities for Mental Patients in India

1. Government Hospital for Mental Care
   Waltair, Visakhapatnam, 530 003
   Andhra Pradesh
2. Institute of Mental Health
   Erragadda, Hyderabad, 500 018
   Andhra Pradesh
3. Mental Hospital
   Tezpur, Darrang, 784 001
   Assam
4. Ranchi Mansik Arogyashala,
   Kanke, Ranchi, 834 006
   Bihar

5. Central Institute of Psychiatry
   Kanke, Ranchi, 834 006
   Bihar
6. Davis Institute of Neuro-Psychiatry
   Boreya Road, Kanke,
   Ranchi, 834 007
   Bihar
7. Mental Hospital,
   Shahibag Road,
   Ahmedabad, 380 004
   Gujarat
8. Mental Hospital
   Karelibaug
   Vadodara, 390 018
   Gujarat
9. Mental Hospital
   Jamnagar, 361 008
   Gujarat
10. Mental Hospital
    Bhuj-Kutch, 370 001
    Gujarat
11. Kasturba Mental Hospital
    Maroli, Tal-Navasari
    Valsad, 396 436
    Gujarat
12. Mental Institution
    Kalawada Rajkot, 360 001
    Gujarat
13. Government Hospital for Psychiatric Diseases
    Jammu, 180 001
    Jammu-Kashmir
14. Government Hospital for Psychiatric Diseases
    Rainaware, Kathi Darwaza
    Srinagar, 190 003
    Jammu and Kashmir
15. National Institute of Mental Health and Neurosciences
    Bengaluru, 560 029
    Karnataka
16. Karnataka Institute of Mental Health
    Dharwad, 580 008
    Karnataka

17. Government Mental Hospital
    Thiruvananthapuram, 680 004
    Kerala
18. Government Mental Hospital
    Calicut, Kozhikode, 673 016
    Kerala
19. Government Mental Hospital
    Thrissur, 680 004,
    Kerala
20. Mental Hospital
    Indore, 452 003
    Madhya Pradesh
21. Mental Hospital
    Gwalior, 474 003
    Madhya Pradesh
22. Central Mental Hospital
    Yervada, Pune, 411 006
    Maharashtra
23. N M Mental Hospital
    Thane, 400 601
    Maharashtra
24. Mental Hospital
    Chhindwara Road, Nagpur, 440 013
    Maharashtra
25. Mental Hospital
    Ratnagiri, 415 612
    Maharashtra
26. Kripamayee Institute for Mental Health
    Miraj, PO, Wanleswadi, Sangli, 416 414
    Maharashtra
27. Mental Hospital,
    Jail Colony, Kohima, 797 001
    Nagaland
28. Mental Health Institute
    SCB Medical College Hospital
    Cuttack, 753 071
    Orissa
29. Mental Hospital (Psychiatric Centre)
    Janta Colony, Jaipur, 302 004
    Rajasthan
30. Punjab Mental Hospital
    Amritsar, 143 001
    Punjab

31. Mental Hospital (Psychiatric Centre)
    Shastri Nagar, Jodhpur, 342 001
    Rajasthan
32. Institute of Mental Health
    Kilpauk, Chennai, 600 010
    Tamil Nadu
33. Mental Hospital
    Agra, 282 002
    Uttar Pradesh
34. Mental Hospital
    Bareilly, 243 001
    Uttar Pradesh
35. Mental Hospital
    Varanasi, 221 002
    Uttar Pradesh
36. Nur Manzil Psychiatric Centre,
    Lal Bagh, Lucknow, 226 001
    Uttar Pradesh
37. Mental Observation Ward
    7, DL Khan Road, Bhawanipur
    Kolkata, 700 025
    West Bengal
38. Hospital for Mental Diseases
    18, gobra Roa, Kolkata, 700 046
    West Bengal
39. Lumbini Park Mental Hospital
    115, Girindra Sarkar Bose Road, Kolkata, 700 039
    West Bengal
40. Duttanagar Mental Health Centre
    Dutta Nagar, Kolkata, 700 077
    West Bengal
41. Mental Hospital
    Mankundu, Hooghly, 712 103
    West Bengal
42. Sarkarpol Mental Hospital
    PO Maheshtala, 24 Parganas, 700 141
    West Bengal
43. Mental Hospital
    PO Berhampur, Murshidabad, 742 101
    West Bengal

44. Hospital for Mental Diseases
    GT Road, Shahdara
    Delhi, 110 032
45. Mental Hospital
    Institute of Psychiatry and Human Behavior
    Altinho, Panaji, 403 001
    Goa, Daman, and Diu.

APPENDIX IV: SUMMARY OF PSYCHIATRIC CLASSIFICATION; ICD-10 (WHO)

Organic, Including Symptomatic, Mental Disorders

F00 Dementia in Alzheimer's disease
F01 Vascular dementia
F02 Dementia in other diseases classified elsewhere
F03 Unspecified dementia
F04 Organic amnesic syndrome, not induced by alcohol and other psychoactive substances
F05 Delirium, not induced by alcohol and other psychoactive substances
F06 Other mental disorders due to brain damage and dysfunction and physical disease
F07 Personality and behavioral disorders due to brain disease damage and dysfunction
F09 Unspecified organic or symptomatic mental disorder.

Mental and Behavioral Disorders Due to Psychoactive Substance Use

F10 Mental and behavioral disorders due to use of alcohol
F11 Mental and behavioral disorders due to use of opioids
F12 Mental and behavioral disorders due to use of cannabinoids
F13 Mental and behavioral disorders due to use of sedatives or hypnotics
F14 Mental and behavioral disorders due to use of cocaine
F15 Mental and behavioral disorders due to use of other stimulants, including caffeine
F16 Mental and behavioral disorders due to use of hallucinogens
F17 Mental and behavioral disorders due to use of tobacco
F18 Mental and behavioral disorders due to use of volatile solvents
F19 Mental and behavioral disorders due to multiple drug use and use of other psychoactive substances.

Schizophrenia, Schizotypal and Delusional Disorders

F20 Schizophrenia
F21 Schizotypal disorder
F22 Persistent delusional disorders
F23 Acute and transient psychotic disorders
F24 Induced delusional disorder
F25 Schizoaffective disorders
F28 Other nonorganic psychotic disorders
F29 Unspecified nonorganic psychosis.

Mood (Affective) Disorders

F30 Manic episode
F31 Bipolar affective disorder
F32 Depressive episode
F33 Recurrent depressive disorder
F34 Persistent mood (affective) disorders
F35 Other mood (affective) disorders
F39 Unspecified mood (affective) disorder.

Neurotic, Stress-Related and Somatoform Disorders

F40 Phobic anxiety disorders
F41 Other anxiety disorders
F42 Obsessive-compulsive disorder
F43 Reaction to severe stress, and adjustment disorders
F44 Dissociative (conversion) disorders
F45 Somatoform disorders
F48 Other neurotic disorders.

Behavioral Syndromes Associated with Physiological Disturbances and Physical Factors

F50 Eating disorders
F51 Nonorganic sleep disorders
F52 Sexual dysfunction not caused by organic disorder or disease
F53 Mental and behavioral disorders associated with the puerperium, not elsewhere classified
F54 Psychological and behavioral factors associated with disorders or disease classified elsewhere
F55 Abuse of non-dependence producing substances
F59 Unspecified behavioral syndromes associated with physiological disturbances and physical factors.

Disorders of Adult personality and Behavior

F60 Specific personality disorders
F61 Mixed and other personality disorders
F62 Enduring personality changes not attributable to brain damage and disease
F63 Habit and impulse disorders
F64 Gender identity disorders

F65 Disorders of sexual preference

F66 Psychological and behavioral disorders associated with sexual development and orientation

F68 Other disorders of adult personality and behavior

F69 Unspecified disorder of adult personality and behavior.

Mental Retardation

F70 Mild mental retardation

F71 Moderate mental retardation

F72 Severe mental retardation

F73 Profound mental retardation

F78 Other mental retardation

F79 Unspecified mental retardation.

Disorders of Psychological Development

F80 Specific developmental disorders of speech and language

F81 Specific developmental disorders of scholistic skills

F82 Specific developmental disorder of motor function

F83 Mixed specific developmental disorders

F84 Pervasive developmental disorders

F88 Other disorders of psychological development

F89 Unspecified disorder of psychological development.

Behavioral and Emotional Disorders with Onset Usually Occurring in Childhood and Adolescence

F90 Hyperkinetic disorders

F91 Conduct disorders

F92 Mixed disorders of conduct and emotions

F93 Emotional disorders with onset specific to childhood

F94 Disorders of social functioning with onset specific to childhood and adolescence

F95 Tic disorders

F98 Other behavioral and emotional disorders with onset usually occurring in childhood and adolescence.

Unspecified Mental Disorder

F99 Mental disorder not otherwise specified.

Glossary

Anhedonia: Inability to experience pleasure in any activity.

Abreaction: A treatment procedure whereby repressed painful experiences are voluntarily recalled to awareness. This ventilation gives therapeutic effect.

Addiction: Irresistible craving for drugs and alcohol which, if withdrawn, produce acute physical and psychological disturbances. The term nowadays used is *drug dependence.*

Affect: A person's emotional feeling and its outward manifestation.

Affective disorder: A psychological disorder in which a disturbance of affect (mood) is predominant. Includes depression and mania.

Adaptation: Excessive motor activity with a feeling of inner tension.

Agoraphobia: Fear of going out alone and of being in a crowded place, fear of open places.

Akathisia: A state of motor restlessness; unable to sit or stand quietly in one place, often seen as a side-effect of some antipsychotics.

Alcoholics Anonymous (AA): Groups of former or ex-alcoholics, who meet to assist other alcoholics through personal and group support.

Ambivalence: The coexistence of two opposing drives, desires, feelings or emotions towards the same person, object or goal; a conflict to do or not to do.

Amnesia: Pathological loss of memory; forgetting may be organic, emotional or mixed origin.

Anorexia nervosa: A psychological disorder marked by severe and prolonged inability to eat, with marked weight loss, amenorrhea and other symptoms; commonly seen in girls and young women.

Anxiety: A feeling of apprehension or tension caused by anticipating an external or internal danger.

Apathy: A mood state—lack of emotional feeling. Commonly seen in schizophrenics.

Attention: The ability to focus on an activity.

Automatism: Undirected behavior that is not consciously controlled, as seen in complex partial seizure (temporal lobe epilepsy).

Autistic thinking: Preoccupations totally removing a person from reality.

Autism: A withdrawn mental state. The person turns away from the outside world and becomes self-absorbed.

Aversion therapy: A type of behavior therapy where a patient's undesirable behavior is associated with unpleasant painful stimulus in an effort to eliminate it. Used in alcohol dependence and sexual disorders.

Battered child syndrome: A child abuse disorder—a child who has suffered repeated injuries, often including fractures and neurologic damage at the hands of parents or other relatives or guardians.

Behavior therapy: A psychological method of treatment. The treatment is designed to modify the patient's behavior directly, not bothering about the underlying causes. Based on learning theory.

Bereavement: A term which can apply to any loss, like death of a close relative or loss of a job.

Bestiality: A sexual disorder, having sexual relation with an animal.

Biogenic amines: Biochemical substances present in the brain. They are of interest because of their possible role in brain functioning and activities of the mind. Subdivided into catecholamines (adrenaline, noradrenaline, dopamine) and the indoleamines (serotonin, etc.).

Biofeedback: Involuntary and unconscious physiological functions are first brought to the awareness of the patient, who is then trained to keep them at a certain level to achieve comfort and to relieve symptoms. A psychological method of treatment.

Bipolar disorder: A mood disorder in which there are both mania and depressive disorder in the same person. Also known as manic depressive psychosis (MDP).

Blunted affect: A reduction in emotional expression.

Cataplexy: Sudden but transient loss of general muscle control. Associated with sleep disorders.

Circumstantiality: Diversion of thoughts with eventual return to the central point.

Clang associations: Associations based on the sound of words.

Cognition: The experience of knowing. The mental process of comprehension, judgment, memory and reasoning.

Community psychiatry: The branch of psychiatry dealing with the provision and delivery of an organized program of mental health care to a specified population.

Concentration: The ability to sustain attention.

Condensation: Fusion of various concepts into one.

Confabulation: The unconscious filling of memory gaps by imagined experiences due to memory impairment.

Conflict: A mental struggle that arises from the simultaneous operation of opposing emotions.

Conversion: A mental defense mechanism by which a psychological conflict (anxiety) is converted and expressed in the form of a physical symptom.

Cretinism: A type of mental retardation caused by thyroid deficiency.

Crisis intervention: Brief therapeutic approach to relieve acute emotional problems.

Culture bound syndromes: A group of disturbed behavior that are highly specific to certain cultures.

Cyclothymic personality: A personality characterized by the presence of mood fluctuations, i.e. alternate depression and elation.

Defense mechanism: Unconscious intrapsychic processes serving to provide relief from psychological conflict and anxiety. Also called as mental mechanism, ego defense mechanism.

Deja vu: The feeling that one has experienced before what is occurring for the first time.

Delusion: A false fixed belief not consistent with the patient's cultural or educational background.

Denial: A defense mechanism by which a person does not accept a fact, which is anxiety and conflict producing in nature.

Delirium: An acute organic mental disorder characterized by disturbance of consciousness, disorientation, disturbance in perception and restlessness.

Delirium tremens: An acute organic mental disorder caused by the withdrawal of alcohol. Starts in 24–96 hours. Characterized by disturbance in consciousness, orientation and perception, and associated with increased ANS activity, convulsions, fever, etc. Reversible if taken care of.

Dementia: A chronic organic mental disorder. An irreversible global deterioration of mental functions.

Dependence syndrome: The use of psychoactive substances has a higher priority than other behaviors that once had higher value. There is a desire, often strong and overpowering to take the substance(s) on a continuous or periodic basis.

Depersonalization: One feels that one or a part of the self is altered and not real in some way.

Derealization: The surroundings do not seem real.

Detoxification: Medical management of alcohol withdrawal state.

Displacement: Transferring an unacceptable thought or feeling to another object. A defense mechanism.

Dissociative Disorder: A disorder in which there is a disturbance in the normal integration of awareness of identity, consciousness and memory. A type of hysteria.

Down's syndrome: A mentally retarded condition due to chromosomal abnormality.

Echolalia: Pathological repetition by imitation of the speech of another.

Echopraxia: Pathologic repetition by imitation of the behavior of another.

Edipus complex: Attachment of the child to the parent of the opposite sex, accompanied by envious feelings towards the parent of the same sex. Attachment of a son towards mother.

Ego: Part of the mental apparatus that serves between ID and super ego.

In simple words, ego is the practical mind.

EPS: Extrapyramidal symptoms. Commonly caused by antipsychotic medication in psychiatry. Acute dystonia, akathisia and tardive dyskinesia are the common extrapyramidal symptoms.

Euphoria: An exaggerated feeling of physical and mental well-being not appropriate to the stimuli. A mood state commonly occurring in mania.

Extrovert: An outgoing and sociable person.

Flat affect: There is almost no emotional expression at all. The patient has an immobile face.

Flight of ideas: Rapid shifting of thoughts, often based on stimuli from the external environment.

Fugue: A dissociative state characterized by amnesia and physical flight away from one's usual environment occur in hysteria, depression and in organic disorders.

Generalized anxiety disorder: A neurotic disorder characterized by excessive anxiety and worry, which is generalized.

Genetic counseling: Counseling based on the facts about the role of inherited genes in the production of diseases. It is helpful in the prevention and better understanding of these disorders.

Geriatric psychiatry: A speciality of psychiatry which deals with mental health problems of the elderly.

Hallucination: A perception in any of the senses in the absence of a specific stimulus. It is a perceptual disorder. For example, auditory hallucination.

Halfway home: A transition place between the hospital and home for mentally ill patients, where the improved mentally ill are given rehabilitation.

Hypnosis: An altered state of consciousness induced by suggestion. This can be used as a form of investigation (to bring out the subconscious wishes) and as a treatment method in some neurotic disorders, like hysteria. This is known as hypnotherapy.

Id: An unconscious part of the mind. It acts upon the pleasure principle, i.e. a pleasure seeking mind.

Ideas of reference: When someone has a mistaken idea that people talk about him, point towards him or make fun of him.

Illusion: A perceptual disturbance. A false perception of a real external stimulus. For example, mistaking a rope as a snake.

Insight: Understanding one's own condition. Lack of insight is characteristic of psychosis.

IQ: Intelligence quotient**:** Intelligence of a person measured through psychological testing. Normal IQ is 90–110 IQ, below 70 denotes mental retardation.

Introvert: A reserved, asocial person.

Jamais vu: The illusion of failure to recognize a familiar situation.

Kleptomania: Compulsion to steal.

Korsakoff's psychosis: A disorder of central nervous system seen in chronic alcoholism. It is due to lack of vitamin B_1 characterized by confabulation and grossly impaired memory.

Labile affect: Rapidly shifting emotions; unstable.

La belle indifference: Seen in hysteria, where certain patients show an inappropriate and lack of concern about their disability.

Lesbianism: Homosexuality in women.

Libido: Psychic drive or energy usually associated with sexual instinct.

Loosening of association: A thinking disturbance, in which thinking becomes diffuse and vague and the associations found to be irrelevant and fail to have an adequate communication with others.

LSD (Lysergic acid diethylamide): A potent drug that produces psychotic symptoms and behavior. An addictive drug.

Mania: A mood disorder characterized by excessive happiness, hyperactivity, agitation and increased thinking and speaking.

Malingering: Deliberate simulation or exaggeration of an illness or disability that is in fact is non-existent or minor.

Manic depressive psychosis: Older terminology for bipolar mood disorder.

Marital counseling; A treatment modality whose goal is to lessen problems of married couples.

Masochism: Pleasure derived from physical or psychological pain inflicted on self.

McNaughton's rule: A rule governing criminal responsibility. A person is not responsible for a crime if the accused was suffering from a disease of the mind as not knowing the nature and quality of the act; or if he did not know what he had done was right or wrong.

Mental retardation: Significantly below average intellectual functioning evident in the developmental period and characterized by impairment in learning, social and adaptive skills.

Mental health: The capacity of an individual to form harmonious relationships with others .

Mental mechanism: Refer defense mechanism.

Mental status examination: The process of estimating psychological and behavioral function by observing the patient, eliciting his subjective description and by questioning the patient.

Milieu therapy: A type of therapy in which the attitudes and behavior of staff of a treatment service and the activities prescribed for the patient are determined by what the patient's emotional and interpersonal needs are. (Syn: therapeutic community).

Minnesota multiphasic personality inventory (MMPI): An inventory to determine personality structure.

Mood: An internal emotional state of an individual.

Mongolism: Refer Down's syndrome.

Munchausen syndrome: A rare, difficult to treat disorder where sufferers habitually attempt to hospitalize themselves with self-inflicted pathology.

Narcissism: Self-love, derived from Narcissus—a figure in Greek mythology who fell in love with his own reflection.

Narcoanalysis: A procedure by which a chemical is introduced to a person (e.g. slow IV injection of pentathol), while encouraging him/her to ventilate the unconscious desires and motives which he/she cannot recollect during conscious state. A therapeutic and a diagnostic procedure commonly used in neurotic disorders.

Narcolepsy: Uncontrollable brief episodes of sleep associated with sleep paralysis and hallucinations.

Negativism: A motiveless resistance to all commands. Commonly seen in catatonic schizophrenia.

Neologism: A word newly coined, or an everyday word used in special way. Coining new words is seen in schizophrenia.

Neurosis: A neurotic disorder is a psychiatric disorder in which the patient has insight into the illness. Only a part of his personality is involved. It is considered to be less severe than psychosis.

Neuroleptic: A psychotropic drug which is antipsychotic in action.

Nihilistic delusion: The delusional belief that others, oneself or the world do not exist.

Nightmare: A sleep disorder characterized by mild anxiety and autonomic reactions, with good recall of dreams.

Nominal aphasia: Difficulty in naming objects.

Norepinephrine: The neurohormone of the peripheral sympathetic nervous system. A neurotransmitter.

Obsessions: Repetitive, senseless thoughts recognized by the patient as being irrational that can, at least initially, be resisted unsuccessfully. The person feels it as absurd, and wants to avoid; but is not able to.

Obsessive compulsive disorder: A neurotic disorder characterized by unwanted thoughts, images or ideas that the individual is unable to stop. He has compulsive acts to minimize this.

Organic mental disorder: Any mental disorder associated with or caused by a disturbance in the physiologic functioning of the brain at any level of organization, structural, hormonal, biochemical, electrical, etc.

Occupational therapy: A therapy that utilizes purposeful activities as a means of altering the course of illness.

Orgasm: Peak reaction to sexual stimulation accompanied by a release of sexual tension.

Panic attack: Acute, episodic intense anxiety attacks with or without physiological symptoms.

Paranoid: An adjective applied to individuals who are oversuspicious.

Paranoid delusion: A firm, unshakable belief that others are trying to harm the self.

Paranoid schizophrenia: A sub-type of schizophrenia, characterized by persecutory delusions, delusions of reference. It is the most common type of schizophrenia.

Parasuicide (deliberate self-harm): Any act deliberately undertaken by a person which mimics the act of suicide, but which does not result in a 'fatal' outcome.

Parkinson's disease: A basal ganglia disorder characterized by involuntary tremors, rigidity of muscles, and slowing of movements.

Passivity phenomenon: The delusional belief that an external agency is controlling aspects of self.

Personality: The characteristic way in which a person behaves. The total qualities of an individual.

Petit mal: Minor, non-convulsive epileptic seizures without loss of control.

Perseveration: Persistent continuation of a line or thought or activity once it is stopped clinically; inappropriate repetition.

Pellagra: A vitamin B_6 (Niacin) deficiency manifested by mental symptoms and impaired thinking, diarrhea and dermatitis.

Personality disorders: Deeply organized and enduring behaviour patterns, generally lifelong in duration, mostly maladaptive.

Phobia: A persistent, irrational fear of an activity, object or situation leading to avoidance of it.

Physical dependence: An adaptive state in which intense physical disturbance occurs when the administration of a psychoactive substance is suspended or withdrawn.

Phenothiazine: A group of psychotropic drugs that are used to control psychotic symptoms.

Phenylketonuria: A genetic metabolic disturbance that is treatable when detected in infancy. Untreated, the condition leads to severe mental retardation.

Pick's disease: A presenile degenerative disease of the brain affecting the frontal lobe. A type of dementia.

Play therapy: A treatment technique utilizing the child's play as a medium of instruction for expression and communication between patient and therapist.

Premenstrual syndrome: Also called late luteal dysphoric disorder: There is a recurrence of emotional, physical and behavioral symptoms occurring regularly during the menstrual cycle.

Primary delusion: A delusion arising fully formed without any previous event.

Posturing: An inappropriate or bizarre bodily posture adopted continuously over a long period. A common symptom seen in catatonic schizophrenia.

Projection: A defense mechanism in which repressed thoughts and wishes are attributed to other people or objects.

Pseudodementia: Similar clinically to dementia, but has a non-organic cause, e.g. depression, reversible.

Psychological dependence: A psychoactive substance (addictive drug) produces a feeling of satisfaction and a psychological drive that requires periodic or continuous administration of the substance to produce pleasure or to avoid the psychological discomfort of its absence.

Psychosis: A psychotic disorder in which the patient does not have insight and his personality is distorted. A major mental disorder.

Psychology: The science investigating the behavior of mental and emotional life.

Psychoanalysis: A psychological theory of the human development and behavior, a method of research and a system of psychotherapy.

Psychodrama: A technique of group psychotherapy in which the individuals express their own or assigned emotional problems.

Psychometry: The science of testing and measuring mental and psychological ability, efficiency, potentials and functioning. Also known as psychological testing.

Psychomotor epilepsy: Recurrent, periodic disturbance, originating in the temporal lobe, of behavior during which the patient carries out movements that are repetitive and automatic in character.

Psychopathology: The study of significant causes and processes in the development of mental disorders.

Psychosurgery: Surgical interventions to modify or alter disturbances of behavior, or thought content.

Psychopathic personality: An informal term for an antisocial personality, where individuals are loveless and guiltless.

Psychotherapy: A procedure carried out by a therapist trained in psychiatry, to treat mental, emotional and psychosomatic illness through a therapeutic relationship with the patient.

Rapport: The feeling of harmonious accord and sympathy that contributes to the patient's confidence. Establishing a meaningful conversation.

Rationalization: A defense mechanism in which the individual attempts to justify or make consciously tolerable by plausible means and behavior.

Reaction formation: A defense mechanism wherein attitudes and behavior are adopted that are opposite of impulses the individual harbors.

Regression: A defense mechanism in which there is a return to an earlier stage of development.

Rehabilitation: That process which attempts to benefit a mentally ill person to bring him as near as possible to his original state. It is a method of making a sick person self sufficient inspite of his disability.

Remission: Recovery from an illness.

Rorschach test: A projective test to identify ego function and personality conflicts which consists of 10 ink blots.

Sadism: Pleasure derived from inflicting physical or psychological pain on others.

Schizoid Personality: A personality disorder characterized by shyness, oversensitivity and preferring to be alone.

Schizophrenia: A large group of disorders usually of psychotic proportion, characterized by disturbance in thought, mood and behavior.

Serotonin: A neurotransmitter found in the central nervous system and implicated in mood disorders.

Social phobia: A term used when a student in the early elementary grades without any apparent reason, refuses to go to school.

Somatization disorder: A neurotic disorder characterized by multiple physical complaints without a known organic cause.

Status epilepticus: Continuous epileptic seizures without regaining complete consciousness in between.

Stupor: A state in which the individual does not react to his surroundings and appears to be unaware of them. Commonly seen in catatonic and depressive disorders.

Subconscious: Used to include the preconscious and the unconscious states of the mind.

Suggestion: The process of influencing an individual to accept less critically an idea or belief induced by the therapist.

Simple phobia: Fear of discrete objects (e.g. spiders) or situations.

Social phobia: Fear of going out to public places or to crowded places.

Somnambulism: Sleep walking.

Tardive dyskinesia: Untoward effect, appearing after long-term use of antipsychotic drugs with muscle involvement around the face, neck, and trunk.

Temporal lobe epilepsy: Refer psychomotor epilepsy.

Thematic apperception test (TAT): A projective test, consisting of 30 cards to identify personality conflicts and defensive structure.

Token economy: Conditioned reinforcers like tokens, points or credits given to the patient when they engage in deviant behavior. Tokens are exchanged as positive reinforcers. Commonly used as a behavior modification technique in chronic schizophrenia and mental retardation.

Toxic psychosis: A psychosis resulting from the poisonous effect of chemicals, drugs and metabolic state.

Tension: An unpleasant increase in psychomotor activity.

Thought block: A sudden interruption in the thought process.

Thought insertion: The delusional belief that thoughts are being put into one's mind.

Thought broadcast: The delusional belief that one's thoughts are being broadcast and read by others.

Transvestism: Sexual pleasure derived from dressing in the clothing of the opposite sex.

Transference: The unconscious process in which emotions and attitudes experienced in childhood are transferred to the therapist. Emphasized in psychoanalytic therapy.

Tolerance: The desired central nervous system effect of a psychoactive substance diminishes with repeated use, so that increasing quantity is necessary to achieve the same effect.

Unconscious: That part of the mind of which the content is only rare subject to awareness.

Undoing: A defense mechanism in which previous thoughts or actions are made not to have occurred.

Unipolar depression: Characterized by recurrent episodes of depression.

Vaginismus: Involuntary spasms of the muscles surrounding the entrance to vagina. A sexual dysfunction in females.

Voyeurism: Sexually motivated and often compulsive interest in watching or looking at others genitals or sexual activity.

Waxy flexibility: Present in catatonic schizophrenia, in which the patient's arm or leg remains passively in an awkwardly position.

Wechsler adult intelligence scale (WAIS): A test for assessing intellectual functioning thought process and ego-functioning.

Wernicke-Korsakoff's syndrome: A disorder of central nervous system seen in chronic alcoholism, characterized by confusion, delirium, eye movement abnormalities, incordination, impaired thinking and sensory motor deficits.

Withdrawal state: Physical and mental effects of withdrawing drugs from patients who have become habituated to them.

Index